THE 7 WONDERS OF OLIVE OIL

FAMILIUS

Published by Familius LLC, www.familius.com

Familius books are available at special discounts for bulk purchases, whether for sales promotions or for family or corporate use. For more information, contact Familius Sales at 559-876-2170 or email orders@familius.com.

Library of Congress Cataloging-in-Publication Data
2016954732

Print ISBN 9781942934738
Ebook ISBN 9781944822361
Hardcover ISBN 9781944822378

Printed in the United States of America

Edited by Lindsay Sandberg and Elena Gonzalez
Cover design by David Miles
Book design by Brooke Jorden
Charts and illustrations by Adam Eastburn

10 9 8 7 6 5 4 3 2 1

First Edition

THE 7 WONDERS OF OLIVE OIL

*Stronger Bones, Cancer Prevention,
Higher Brain Function, and Other
Medical Miracles of the Green Nectar*

ALICE ALECH AND CÉCILE LE GALLIARD

DISCLAIMER NOTICE

This book is not intended as a substitute for medical advice. Readers should consult their physician in matters relating to health, especially if the symptoms require medical attention.

The authors would like to point out that the olive oil world, in regards to both business and culture, is a changing one. New information, studies, results, and figures will not be the same in years to come. The authors made every effort to ensure the information in this book was correct at press time. Both the authors and the publisher disclaim any liability caused by error or omission.

Who We Are

We are two olive oil enthusiasts living in different regions in France. Cécile lives in Southwest France, a little less than 100 kilometers from the Spanish border, and Alice lives in a small village in Provence, around 90 kilometers inland from Nice.

We first met on the Internet a few years ago through our writing on olive oil features and stories, Alice through her writing covering olive oil news from France and Cécile on her French blog *Jus d'olive*.

We started sharing our knowledge and resources essentially for our writing, building a strong working relationship before we finally met. The idea of writing this book came one day when it dawned on us that even though the world is slowly recognizing the goodness of olive oil, there is still much to learn. We pooled our knowledge and our expertise, enlisted the help of experts, and embarked on preparing *The 7 Wonders of Olive Oil*. It led us to family farms and research institutions and allowed us to talk to researchers, nutritionists, and chefs.

We, too, had much more to learn about the nutritional secrets of this highly beneficial food.

We hope you enjoy reading this book as much as we did writing it.

Contents

INTRODUCTION

A beautiful French woman, Jeanne Calment, lived to be 122 years old. Toward the end of her life, when asked the secret of her longevity and her relatively youthful appearance, she had two words: "olive oil." This supercentenarian French lady was alert right until the end of her life.

Olive oil, our gift from Mother Nature, has always been praised by dietitians, nutritionists, and medical researchers worldwide. They say, "Olive oil is good for your health and well-being." Today, consumers are more health conscious. More curious than ever, they want to understand the medical research behind the health benefits, they need to know how they should be taking this monounsaturated fat, and, most importantly, they want to understand why they should include extra-virgin olive oil in their daily diets. Countless studies on the different health benefits of olive oil have been discussed over the years, and scientists are constantly discovering more. We could not include all these research projects, but what we discuss in *The 7 Wonders of Olive Oil* is based on interviews with the researchers involved in the studies, published research carried out in laboratory studies, randomized clinical trials, and observational studies. Without being too academic, we describe health conditions and show the extraordinary work and positive results that scientists have achieved so far.

In order to fully grasp the work of these researchers, consumers need to understand olive oil. What you'll find in *7 Wonders*—in addition to the astounding health benefits of olive oil—is a comprehensive guide to extra-virgin olive oil, how it's made, and the different types of olive oil available, as well as tips on storing and cooking.

Excellent olive oil comes from excellent fruit. This is one of the first things we as olive oil enthusiasts have come to appreciate more and more. We also realize that even though olive oil is one of the oldest products in history, not many people understand the basics of olive oil production, what a well-balanced extra-virgin olive oil should taste like, or, equally important, the practical side of buying, storing, and cooking with olive oil. This book answers all of these questions.

The 7 Wonders of Olive Oil has three major sections:

Part I looks at the history of the Mediterranean culture, followed by a description of olive oil processing. It covers harvesting and milling, looking at some of the choices modern-day producers have to face—questions such as when the best time to pick the olives is and whether or not producers should filter the oil. We conclude this section by discussing the complicated business of fats and how olive oil is different from other oils.

Part II is a more in-depth study of the healthful characteristics of olive oil. It describes the research into the nutritional, medicinal, and cosmetic values of olive oil. We show you through scientific discoveries that olive oil is a therapeutic agent fighting diseases such as cancer, diabetes, and Alzheimer's and why it is so important to incorporate this gift from Mother Nature into our daily diets for health and beauty.

Dr. Oreste Gualillo, one of the scientists whose findings contributed to this book, sums up the value of this research:

Natural products have been used for thousands of years for the treatment of many diseases and pathological conditions. Thus, nature is a vast source of bioactive molecules from terrestrial and marine environments. Many of these natural products have gone on to become current drug candidates. The era of modern pharmacology is the result of man experimenting by trial and error for hundreds of centuries through palatability trials or untimely deaths, searching for available foods for the treatment of diseases.

What he means by this is that Nature has been providing the necessary ingredients for healthful living since the beginning. We are just using the elements that she offers to us to find healing.

In Part III, we offer you practical advice and information to help you figure out what it is that you should look for when purchasing olive oil. Food magazines and cookbooks say you should be using olive oil in the kitchen, but the choices in the supermarkets these days are overwhelming. As consumers, you want to understand the tricky business of labeling, especially when olive oil quality and authenticity are being questioned. This final section explains why you should not reject oil just because it causes a sting at the back of your throat and how to store your oil once you buy it.

The olive oil world has changed over the years. Olive oil keeps making the news, attracting the attention of people from all walks of life—from health-conscious baby boomers to nutritionists and medical experts.

"Let food be thy medicine and medicine be thy food," said Hippocrates, fifth-century Greek physician and philosopher, considered by some the "father of medicine." How right he was! But today, we are afflicted by a plethora of noncommunicable diseases, the leading cause of death worldwide and a new challenge for all global health policies. If only we could put Hippocrates's advice into practice.

More than anything, we want this book to be inspiring, to show you that the humble olive fruit produces a most powerful natural oil that can make a significant difference to our health.

PART I

OLIVE OIL:

THE CORNERSTONE OF MEDITERRANEAN HISTORY

According to legend, Zeus, King of the Gods, settled the dispute between Athena, Goddess of Wisdom, and Poseidon, God of the Sea, by asking them to provide a gift to a new city over which they both claimed sovereignty. While Poseidon offered the city a horse laden with weapons and an invincible army of warriors, Athena drew a tree from the ground, an olive tree, to nourish and to heal wounds and ailments—a gift which would last forever. The people declared that the olive tree was more useful to humanity. Hence, the city was named Athens.

All civilizations and religions of the Mediterranean bestowed a spiritual importance upon the olive tree. There are an incredible number of references to olive oil and the olive tree in the religious scriptures of Judaism, Christianity, and Islam. It has been a symbol of peace and abundance to the Greeks and an emblem of benediction to Christians. One of the best-known Biblical references is the olive branch brought to Noah as a symbol of reconciliation between God and mankind and a sign that the flood was over. The Catholic Church uses it widely in its rituals, especially for anointing. In the rabbinic tradition, there is the miracle of the olive oil lamp that illuminated the temple for eight days following the military and spiritual victory of the Jews of Judea even though there was only enough oil to light the temple for one day. The significance of olive oil and its association with light has been perpetuated in the most important Jewish festival of Hanukkah, the Jewish Festival of Lights, by lighting the seven-branch candelabra, the Menorah. In addition, olive oil fuels the lamps of the Shabbat and other ritual celebrations. In the Koran, the olive tree is described as sacred, a symbol of Universal Man. It is compared to the bright light of Allah that illuminates the path of mankind. Even as far to the east as Japan, it is a symbol of social success.

In modern times, the olive branch continues to symbolize peace. The United Nations flag is a good example of the meaning of "holding out an olive branch." It shows a map of the earth framed by olive branches, a symbolic peace surrounding the world. Another present-day symbol is the Great Seal of the United States, which features an eagle holding in the left talon thirteen arrows and in the right one an olive branch. Although the arrows suggest war, the eagle's head is turned toward the olive branch, representing peace.

The origins of the olive tree, when and where it was first cultivated, remain uncertain. Fossilized leaves from the Paleolithic and Neolithic ages were found on the edges of the Sahara and dated as far back as 12,000 BC. However, it was probably first cultivated by man in Asia Minor or on the coast of Lebanon or Palestine between 6000 and 5000 BC. The olive tree and the Mediterranean have always been inseparable; the olive tree has linked the past civilizations, people, cultures, and religions in the region. Scientific evidence proves that olive trees had been growing in Crete as early as 3500 BC, long before spreading to mainland Greece.

As the first civilizations were emerging in the Mediterranean basin and the Middle East, cereals, vines, and olive trees were the top three staple food sources. The first vegetable oils were extracted from olives in the West. (In the East, it was extracted from sesame.)

Extracting these oils required a simple mechanical force easily exerted by humans or animals. Just think: for a long time, these were the only edible oils the people at the time were familiar with.

We find that the first cultivated trees coincide with the birth of the Phoenician, Assyrian, Jewish, Egyptian, and Greek cultures as well as other less studied Mediterranean cultures. The first written documents on the olive tree are Mycenaean clay tablets dating back to the reign of King Minos (2500 BC), which shows how important olive oil was to the Cretan economy.

It is believed that the Phoenicians—the original inhabitants of Phoenicia in what is now Lebanon—were the first people to spread olive-growing culture in 4000 BC. This civilization died out between 1200 and 300 BC. Few records remain of this period, but it seems that the Phoenicians were excellent merchants, artisans, and navigators and that they were the first to disseminate olive growing through their commercial exchanges with Crete, Greece, the Aegean Islands, Italy, and the western part of the Iberian Peninsula. The remains of amphorae (storage jars for transporting food such as oil and wine on long voyages) were found in shipwrecks.

Olive-growing culture spread to Greece via Anatolia (modern day Turkey) before reaching Crete and Egypt and eventually the whole Mediterranean basin. The Greeks brought olive trees to Corsica, Sardinia, Sicily, all of Italy, and France, specifically the city of Marseille in 600 BC. Perhaps most notably, the Greeks spread olive trees to Al Andalus, the modern Andalusia in Spain, which is considered a leader in olive oil production today.

This healthy oil, sometimes called "green gold" or "liquid gold," played a fundamental role in forging the Mediterranean character— the common thread that binds all of its peoples. The culture of olive oil quickly spread to become a prized commercial product for cooking and cosmetics, a fuel for lighting the lamps of cities and temples, and an important part of religious rituals. At the time of Venetian trade, olive oil was highly prized for the manufacture of soap and the treatment of skin. The term "lampante" olive oil comes from the use of olive oils unfit for human consumption but good for lighting lamps.

It was the Roman Empire that introduced technical improvements, developing plantations and olive mills. Olive growing was exported to all the Roman colonies. As a result, the olive tree became a symbol of economic modernity. The precious oil was stored and carried in tall jars called amphorae. You can see just how important the olive oil trade was under Roman rule when you look at the Monte Testaccio in Rome—an ancient landfill site with an enormous pile of oil amphorae. Once the oil was poured out of the amphora pottery, it was sold in the markets of the city and the amphorae were carefully arranged in layers. Over time, the amphorae ended up forming this artificial mountain.

The decline of the Roman Empire in the fifth century and the arrival of the barbarians and the first Arab invasions interrupted the Roman advances in producing olive oil. It was not until the Crusades, specifically during the time that Venetian trade expanded, that production began to develop once more. In 1497, the sea route to India was discovered and olive trees were brought farther east. Similarly, the olive tree also traveled west to Argentina, Peru, Chile, Mexico, and California in the United States. With the discovery of the new world, Venice lost its monopoly and the market was shared by Italy, Greece, and Portugal. Even to this day, the trade and production of olive oil are widely confined to Europe. The European Union is the world's leading producer, accounting for 73 percent of production, and the leading consumer of olive oil, at 63 percent. Spain, Italy, and Greece together account for 97 percent of total olive oil production in the European Union. Olive oil cultivation in the Americas did not reach the same prominence until the twentieth century as public awareness of the goodness of olive oil became widespread.

In recent times and as the thirst for and success of olive oil grew, the need for setting up standards for chemical, physical, and sensory characteristics of olive oil was apparent. The International Olive Council (IOC), an intergovernmental body, was instituted by the United Nations in 1959 in Madrid. It is the world's only institution with the objective of promoting and defending the entire olive oil and table olive industries worldwide. They are involved in supplying aid and advice to growers and millers as well as funding research to improve the quality of olive oil.

It is a complex business as the IOC currently counts a total of forty-three member nations, including the European Union with its twenty-seven member states. These member countries account for 98% of the world's olive oil production. Today, the IOC faces new challenges when it comes to controlling quality. Their duties extend to coping with fraud and harmonizing trade and production as well as protecting the rights of consumers by implementing the agreement signed in 2005 by the member states. One of the main purposes of the agreement is that it standardizes processing controls and labeling by assigning specific names and definitions to the different oils.

Olive oil is one of the most regulated food industry products. The growers and producers put in a lot of effort to make sure that the olive oil that you bring home is full of the seven wonderful traits that make it so healthful. After all stages of development and before bottling, a sample gets sent to the laboratory for careful examination. This involves examining not ten or fifteen but a total of twenty-six physical and chemical parameters, including acidity and sensory tests, both vital for complete evaluation of the oil. The sensory tests are carried out by a panel of eight to twelve experts and can take place in any member country of the International Olive Oil Council. This means that olive oil in Puglia in southern Italy and olive oil in southern Algeria have had the same quality testing measures as enforced by the IOC.

Even non–IOC member countries have their own strict standards. They protect the consumer through commissions, associations, and organizations such as the California Olive Oil Council (COOC) in the United States and the North American Olive Oil Association (NAOOA). Two other notable organizations are the Australian Olive Association (AOA), promoting olive oil from Australia, and the Association Française Interprofessionnelle de l'Olive (AFIDOL) from France.

But why does olive oil need such high standards and regulation? You might wonder if it's even worth all the fuss. In 2013, the United Nations Educational Scientific and Cultural Organization (UNESCO) recognized the Mediterranean diet as part of the intangible cultural heritage of Spain, Portugal, Morocco, Italy, Greece, Cyprus, and Croatia. These countries' intangible heritage, normally associated with natural wonders, monuments, and temples, now included a different culture: an eating pattern which incorporated olive oil as the main source of fat.

This served as an important international recognition of olives and olive oil. However, this recognition came in a worldwide culture that used olive oil very little. Since the beginning of the industrial era, other refined vegetable oils were on the market, which seemed a more profitable venture in Western countries. As a result, very little olive oil is now consumed. Palm oil and soybean oil are the world's most consumed vegetable oils, at 32% and 28%, respectively, followed by rapeseed oil at 16% and sunflower oil at 8%.

International Olive Council Executive Director, M. Abdellatif Ghedira, stated:

> In recent years, world olive oil production has increased considerably, but olive oil still only accounts for just over 3% of all the vegetable oils produced in the world. So, of course, there is room for expanding this percentage share. World consumption of olive oil can only go upwards: it is so healthy and so delicious that I am very optimistic about its future.

And he is correct! New producers have entered the market, including the United States, Canada, Australia, Brazil, and Japan. Today, olive trees are grown and olive oil is produced on five continents. It was only in 2008 that the olive oil industry took off in India, but olive trees are now cultivated successfully in the desert region of Rajasthan. The first fruit should soon appear, a good thing for the country, which presently imports a total of 2,617 tons of oil, 195 tons of which is virgin olive oil. The new domestic production of olive oil will certainly influence the Indian diet and alter the import of oil.

Still, the market beyond the Mediterranean basin is still in its infancy. The Chinese market, attracted to the western lifestyle, imports more and more olive oil each year; 14,000 tons were imported in 2010. Another burgeoning market is the United States, where consumption reached 248,000 tons in 2006, ranking it the world's second olive oil consumer after Europe and also the leading importer.

The last thirty years have seen a worldwide shift in consumer habits toward healthier and more natural foods. As a healthy alternative to other fats, the average annual olive oil consumption has already reached 2.8 million tons and will reach 3 million tons in 2016.

We asked Abdellatif Ghedira what the major advances have been these ten last years. This is what he said: "Agriculturally speaking, I think the biggest changes in the last decade have been—amongst other things—that cultural practices have improved and irrigated acreage has increased. On the consumption side, world imports of olive oil have expanded by 29% during the same period. This means that olive oil is no longer a local product but has become a global product that reaches every corner of the world."

Let's not forget the impact on health over the years. Almost 2,500 years ago, Hippocrates called olive oil "the great healer" and described at least sixty medical conditions that could be treated with olive oil, including skin conditions, wounds, burns, and other ailments. Today, researchers are delving more and more into the health benefits of the green nectar.

The ancient Greeks cherished olive oil; for them, it was a necessity for daily sustenance. Sadly, over time, olive oil lost its special place as the people turned to other sources of fat. However, olive oil was not the only fat rejected and misunderstood by consumers and nutritionists. Fats in general were seen as unhealthy, as causing heart attacks and leading to obesity; they were the first thing to eliminate if you wanted to go on a diet. Thankfully, since the 2000s, things have changed. New scientific studies are proving the health benefits of virgin olive oils and the importance of fatty acids in our daily diet. As we discuss the seven wonders of olive oil, we'll share with you some of the studies that prove its healing properties.

Today, olive oil has opened up a whole new world of sensory pleasures, taking cooking to new heights, which will no doubt continue to give olive oil a well-deserved and special role in our cuisine.

UNDERSTANDING FATS

Fat is often considered the prime suspect for weight gain, but the body needs a certain amount and certain kinds of fat to survive.

The human body requires energy to function correctly, energy which comes from the nutrients in the food we eat. Food gets processed by our digestive system and then goes into our bodies through our circulatory system, traveling to our cells and supplying them with proteins, carbohydrates, and lipids, or fats.

Fats are a necessity for the correct functioning of our bodies. They provide a rich source of energy. They supply the necessary calories used directly by the body for growth and general functioning. To respond to all their fundamental needs throughout the day, a healthy adult man or woman, doing regular physical exercise with a daily energy intake of 2000 kilocalories, should ideally obtain 55% of their energy from carbohydrates, 15% from proteins, and, finally, a minimum of 30% from lipids. Fats, a rich source of energy, come from certain foods, particularly butter, milk, vegetable oils, meat, and cheese.

Fatty acids are classed as the simplest lipids because of their structure. They serve as fuel for our muscles and help to build cell membranes. Certain fatty acids are termed "essential" because the body does not produce them—we have to consume them in food.

There are three main types of fatty acids: saturated, monounsaturated, and polyunsaturated. They are similar in that they have similar chemical structures and they contain a chain of carbon atoms bonded with hydrogen atoms. However, all three have different roles to play in the human body and have complex differences in form and function.

DIFFERENT FAMILIES OF FATTY ACID AND RECOMMENDED NUTRIENTS INTAKES (RNI)

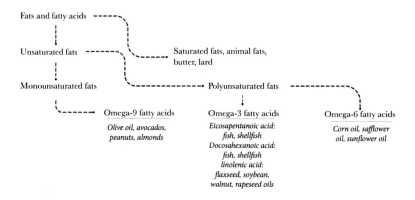

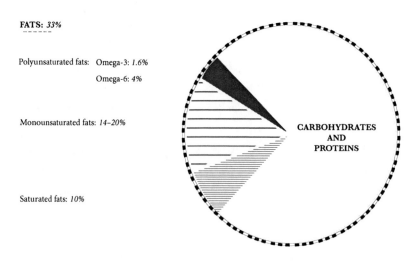

How are they different?

- Saturated fats are solid at room temperature because they are "saturated" with hydrogen molecules.

- Monounsaturated fats—often classed as good fats—are liquid at room temperature because they contain fewer hydrogen atoms.

- Polyunsaturated fats—also considered good fats and liquid at room temperature—are broken into two main types: omega-3 fatty acids and omega-6 fatty acids.

Oleic acid is one of the main types of monounsaturated fatty acids. It can be found directly in food, especially in olives and in olive oil, as well as in rapeseed oil, peanut oil, nuts, almonds, avocados, goose fat, meat, oily fish, and, to a lesser amount, processed meats. Products containing oleic acid carry the name "omega-9" on the food label. Oils containing monounsaturated fats are usually liquid at room temperature but start turning solid when chilled. Monounsaturated fatty acids protect the heart, playing a fundamental role in preventing cardiovascular diseases. They affect the cholesterol levels in the blood and are known to reduce bad cholesterol, or LDL, and to increase good cholesterol, or HDL.

Polyunsaturated fatty acids, commonly referred to as omega-3 and omega-6 acids, deserve special mention. The body does not produce these well-publicized fats; we can get them only from foods, mostly from plant food and certain seafood. That is why they are often called "essential fats." Fatty acids make up 60% of the brain and are necessary for the correct functioning of our gray matter.

Studies on the importance of fatty acids, their role, and the recommended nutritional intake for each family of fatty acids are very recent. In the 1950s, Ancel Keys, an American doctor and researcher, was one of the first to establish a link between our diet and our health.

During the 1950s in the United States, the population and medical professionals were confronted with a major public health concern: the number of deaths from heart attacks was rising continuously. Autopsies revealed the presence of cholesterol in the arteries. Those studies lead to the campaign against cholesterol. Up until then, scientists were convinced that having a diet rich in products of animal origin was the best way to stay in good health. This belief was later rejected by some studies.

It was during this period that Ancel Keys conducted his first survey in Naples, Italy. He discovered that cardiovascular diseases affected the more affluent populations; one of the main differences between the rich and the poor was that the rich ate more meat. It showed a clear connection between the consumption of fats and the risk of death from cardiovascular disease.

Following this first observation, he began, in 1952, to study seven countries. He decided to compare the diet and cardiovascular health of populations in the United States, Finland, Italy, Japan, the Netherlands, Yugoslavia, and Greece; he especially wanted to study those living on the island of Crete. This intriguing study included 13,000 volunteers and lasted twenty-five years. It showed that in the northern nations—Finland, the Netherlands, and the United States—a lot of animal fats were consumed in meat, butter, and cheese, while there was only a small amount of fruits and vegetables consumed. In the southern nations, specifically in Crete, vegetable fats and olive oil were the main fats consumed, together with a healthy intake of nuts, vegetables, fruit, and fish. The results of the study showed that the Cretans presented with the lowest rate of cardiovascular-related deaths—six times lower than the Finns—and enjoyed a lower rate of cancer and greater longevity.

Although Ancel Keys's results and the studies themselves were very heavily criticized in later years, the study of the Cretan diet marked a turning point in the close relationship between our food intake, our health, and the beneficial and protective quality of diets rich in monounsaturated and polyunsaturated fats.

Studies of these differences in types of fatty acids are very recent. Until 2010, people were told to reduce their intake of all fats and to switch to low-fat foods. Since then, however, daily energy intake and the role of fats have been reevaluated. The emphasis today is more on choosing the right fat, creating a shift from a quantitative view of fatty acids to a more qualitative one. The recommended daily intake now varies according to the properties of the fat and the individual's needs.

Dietician, nutritionist, and head of the School of Human Nutrition and Dietetics in Paris Anne-Laure Meunier says that we should consume fats according to our needs, as well as our taste, but warns that we should avoid hydrogenated fats. These fatty acids or trans-fatty acids are processed industrially with high-pressure oxygen; they are the culprits that clog up our cardiovascular system. Meunier, who specializes in obesity in adults, says that a healthier choice would be to opt for virgin oils, which have been pressed or extracted by mechanical means such as "real" butter and "real" cream. She says that we should also consume only what is necessary; although we do need to eat fat, we should aim for good fats and to have them in reasonable quantities.

Large amounts of saturated fatty acids are found in food, but they are also produced by the human body in the liver, the brain, and the adipose tissue (fat cells). Besides being vital sources of energy, saturated fats are also essential for transporting vitamins A, D, E, and K in the body. These vitamins are fat soluble, which means they are carried through the body in oils. Our bodies naturally create these fats to generate energy and transport nutrients, but we need to find the right balance, to get the right ratios of fatty acids for optimum health. Most saturated fatty acids are of animal origins, such as meat from cows, sheep, lambs, and pigs. We find them also in dairy products: butter, fresh cream, whole milk, and cheese. Where we can, limiting these animal products in our diets can help us maintain a healthy balance of saturated fats in our bodies.

Palm oil, soybeans, and coconut oil (plant-based vegetable oils) are also sources of saturated fats. Although the body needs saturated fatty acids, consuming too much only results in an accumulation of bad cholesterol. This is bad news for our bodies, because from that we become overweight and suffer from other related illnesses such as cardiovascular disease, high blood pressure, and heart attacks.

As we search for and select saturated, monounsaturated, and polyunsaturated fats in our food, the first challenge is knowing where to find them. Secondly, they must be in the right proportions. According to the French Agency for Food, Environmental, and Occupational Health and Safety (ANSES), for correctly balanced overall health, the ratio consumed must be 1 to 5: 1 portion of omega-3 acids for every 5 portions of omega-6 acids. Imbalance leads to excess fats stored in the body, causing first weight gain then cardiovascular problems. In France, for example, the ratio of omega-3 acids to omega-6 acids is 1 to 10; in the United States, it is 1 to 40.

Without realizing, we now consume far more omega-6 fatty acids than our grandparents' generation did. Back then, cows simply grazed on grass in the fields and ate hay during the winter. However, the story is different these days. With beef producers focusing more on increased production and maximum profits, cow feed today includes cereals such as corn, sunflower, meal, and soybeans. As a result, all products that we get from cows, such as milk, butter, cheese, and cream, are already naturally enriched with omega-6 acids.

At the same time, there has been an increased consumption of omega-6 type fatty acids due to a rise in direct consumption in the household; changes in production and extraction methods mean that these fatty acids are used to make cheap oils.

We find omega-6 acids in sunflower oil, safflower oil, soybean oil, corn oil, and grapeseed oil, whereas omega-3s come from linseed oil, rapeseed oil, soybean oil, and all oily fish. Some oils such as walnut oil and groundnut oil contain both in large quantities.

While much of the world has consumed increasing amounts of unhealthy fatty acids, there is one notable exception. Since 2010, the Mediterranean diet, which includes the Cretan diet, has been listed as intangible cultural heritage of humanity by UNESCO. The countries that submitted recommendations were Cyprus, Croatia, Spain, Greece, Italy, Morocco, and Portugal. There is no single model of the Mediterranean diet; instead, it is more about the eating habits of these countries bordering the Mediterranean Sea. According to the UNESCO definition, the Mediterranean diet is not only a combination of know-how, rituals, symbols, and traditions but also involves the practice of sitting down to share a meal and consume food together. The act of eating together is a fundamental part of the cultural lifestyle in the Mediterranean basin.

The countries that seem to ascribe to the Mediterranean diet enjoy certain things in common, such as food obtained from livestock, fishing, and agriculture. They also have an abundance of fruits, vegetables, cereals, and olive oil and only moderate consumption of meat, dairy products, and wine. Traditionally, moderation is one of the defining characteristics of the Mediterranean diet.

Meunier concludes: "Based on fish, olive oil, fruits, vegetables, and legumes, the Mediterranean diet has color; it is varied and comes with simple advice that helps to maintain a healthy balance between the different fatty acids."

To conclude, it is all a question of getting the right balance. Saturated, monounsaturated, and polyunsaturated fatty acids all have different functions within the body; they are all vital for the various systems of the body to function. As you come to better understand the characteristics of fats and your own need for the different kinds and quantities, we hope that you are able to enjoy a similarly colorful diet that is balanced and helps you discover the wonders that our foods can provide for us.

FROM OLIVE TO OIL

P roducing oil from the humble olive is an exciting process. For growers and producers striving to get the best extra-virgin oil, it is both a business and a labor of love.

The olive is not an ordinary fruit. You cannot pick it off the tree and eat it; it is so bitter that you would spit it out immediately. But the fruit contains proven health-protective nutrients and organic matter. The challenge for producers is that the fruit also contains a lot of water, which must be extracted before they can obtain the oil.

October is a busy but exciting time for olive oil farmers and producers in Europe. Millers have to make sure their machines are spotlessly clean and in good running condition, ready to wash and process the picked fruit, while farmers lovingly examine their trees every day, checking to see if the olives are ripe enough. The right time for picking olives sparks all sorts of discussions amongst growers; only the best possible olives picked at the right time yield what they are all aiming for: good quality extra-virgin olive oil with excellent flavor, nutritional goodness, and a decent shelf life. After the flowering period, the olives first appear green then change color as they ripen from rosy to mauve. The color of the fruit on the outside corresponds to the different chemical changes taking place within. It's difficult to extract oil from green olives, and they don't give as much oil, but olives that are too ripe lack polyphenols and become less stable with time.

When nurtured appropriately, picked at the right time, and processed with precision, good-quality olive oil will have high levels of polyphenols, the phytonutrients in plants that are recognized scientifically as potent antioxidants. Olive oil contains a multitude of polyphenols; these are the health components that scientists love—they are extra-virgin olive oil's most powerful weapon for protecting the body and preventing diseases.

Some farmers pick their olives by hand, while others use a machine. In the past, European farmers would start the harvest in December and continue slowly until February the following year when the fruit was well and truly black in color and the oil easy to extract. By then, however, the intrinsic qualities of the oil had reduced considerably in the overripe fruit.

Things have changed significantly over the years, with farmers striving to improve quality rather than quantity. Following the advice of the IOC and other research centers, they now harvest olives earlier, achieving more nourishing oil with all the desired organoleptic properties: taste, odor, color, and texture. The tendency these days is to pick olives while the skin is between green and mauve and the pulp still green. In Mediterranean countries, this usually happens between the second week in October and the second week in November. Experts at the IOC say this is the best time to get the maximum nutrients and aroma from the fruit. Most importantly, this is when the fruit is full of polyphenols and antioxidants. Once picked and collected, the olives must be thoroughly washed, dried, and weighed at the mill.

Though the methods vary with time and technology, making olive oil always involves picking good fruit, crushing the fruit, and separating out the water. With proper treatment of the olives, the resulting oil is beautiful and has incredible health benefits!

The Traditional Approach

Though technology has advanced to allow farmers to produce good, clean olive oil in a short time, we think it is important to remember the heritage of the olive press and the traditional method to crush olives. The idea of a donkey or a mule turning a great stone mill might seem a bit far-fetched, but that's how they crushed olives thousands of years ago.

The millstone was set in a trough where farmers poured the cleaned olives. As the millstone rotated, it broke, crushed, and ground the cleaned olives to a thick paste. The mixing or malaxing stage followed—a period of about an hour of continued grinding that made sure the olives were fully ground and allowed the fruit enzymes to develop.

After milling and malaxing, mill workers would spread the thick paste onto fiber discs, which look like mats placed one on top of the other. These stacks of mats then went into a vertical hydraulic press and were pressed; several hundred pounds of pressure applied squeezed everything to the maximum. Fifty-six kilograms of ground olives stacked and pressed would yield a little over seven liters of oil.

Olive oil processed this traditional way is sometimes referred to as cold-pressed olive oil, meaning no heat or chemicals have been added to alter the taste. You will, however, find labels saying "cold press," "first press," or even "first cold press" on packaging today when the oils were made using the centrifugal method.

Farmers with small quantities of oil still use this traditional system, especially in rural areas of France, Spain, Italy, Morocco, and Tunisia.

The main disadvantage of the traditional system, however, is the danger of oxidation and fermentation because the process is slow and discontinuous. Processing does not take place immediately after harvesting, and waiting during the processing cycle exposes the olive paste to oxygen and light.

The modern mill is certainly not as romantic, and gone is the charm of bygone days, but with the modern crusher, mixer, extractor, and stainless-steel vats, fewer workers are necessary to oversee the extracting process, meaning less worry for the mill owners, especially when they have vast quantities of oil to process. Traditional producers argue that the slow mixing of oil and water gives them better quality and quantity than modern mills.

Not surprisingly, the tastes using these two methods are quite different. Traditionally processed oil is fruity, less bitter, and slightly herbaceous but complex. Oils processed by the modern centrifugal system are more herbaceous, robust, bitter, and pungent with an aroma reminding us of fresh vegetables.

Clearly, production methods have become more sophisticated over the years, more challenging for both the small and large olive oil producer. With growing public awareness of olive oil today, keeping up with new techniques and new developments is essential to producing high-quality olive oil.

The modern methods of processing oil are clearly developed from the traditional methods. After picking the olives, either by hand or by machine, the whole olives are then crushed and ground to form a fine paste, a mixture of fruit and stone. For this process, millers use different types of equipment: the two main types of machines are the modern stainless steel crusher and the more traditional mechanical rollers.

The fruit then needs to be mixed for about thirty to forty minutes at a temperature no higher than 27° C (80° F). Mixing is a critical phase, as this is when the flavor develops. Mixing, sometimes referred to as malaxing, also allows the smaller droplets of oil to mix with the larger ones.

The next step is the separation of the oil from the water and solids. In the past, they called this the first press or cold press because old wooden vertical presses used to be operated with very low temperatures. Often, producers would press the paste a second time to obtain the maximum oil. Although you might still hear these terms, think of them mostly as commercial terms mainly used for marketing olive oil. Modern-day methods are very different.

Today, many mills are equipped with modern centrifuge decanter systems, which use high centrifugal force to allow the water and oil to separate easily. Some producers opt for a three-phase centrifuge system because these machines separate the oil, water, and solids separately, while others prefer a two-phase centrifuge, which separates the oil from the wet paste.

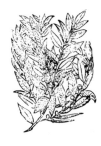

WORLD OLIVE OIL PRODUCTION AND CONSUMPTION

Top Ten Producers of OO in volume (million tons) from 2012–2014

PRODUCTION

	2011 / 2012	2012 / 2013	2013 / 2014
SPAIN	1615,0	1615,0	1615,0
ITALY	399,2	399,2	399,2
GREECE	294,6	294,6	294,6
TURKEY	191,0	191,0	191,0
SYRIA	198,0	198,0	198,0
MOROCCO	120,0	120,0	120,0
TUNISIA	182,0	182,0	182,0
PORTUGAL	76,2	76,2	76,2
ALGERIA	39,5	39,5	39,5
CHILE	21,5	21,5	21,5

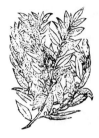

Top Ten Consumers of OO in volume (million tons) from 2012–2014

	CONSUMPTION		
	2011 / 2012	2012 / 2013	2013 / 2014
ITALY	610,0	590,0	600,0
SPAIN	574,0	513,0	580,0
U.S.A.	300,0	293,0	294,0
GREECE	200,0	200,0	185,0
TURKEY	150,0	160,0	150,0
MOROCCO	122,0	129,0	132,0
FRANCE	112,0	97,2	99,6
SYRIA	135,5	135,5	95,0
PORTUGAL	78,0	74,0	74,0
BRAZIL	68,0	73,0	73,0

Harvesting Time in Sunny Spain

In Hellín, Spain, they certainly know how to make fine extra-virgin olive oil, oil that is recognized worldwide.

Two olive growers, Dominguez and Olivares, from a region in the heart of Spain, worked hard at their orchards in 2015, aiming to produce the very best oil they could. Their labor was rewarded. For the first time, their brand Pago de Peñarrubia (made from the delicate Arbequina olive variety) won a gold award at the prestigious New York International Olive Oil Competition (NYIOC) in 2016. More international recognition followed, with silver medals from the Los Angeles International Extra Virgin Olive Oil competition and the Olive Japan International Extra Virgin Olive Oil Competition.

And at home in Spain, they were finalists in the Mario Solinas competition, recognized for the fine flavor of their ripe, fruity extra virgin category for 2016.

This is how they did it:

The region is blessed with great weather; the sun perched high all year round means temperatures of about 35° C (95° F) at the height of the summer season in August—perfect for the magnificent olive trees dotted all around the hillsides.

Their families have been in the business for over a hundred years, striving every year to produce the best-quality olive oil. In the olive oil world, their farms are classed as intensive and super-intensive plantations because of the high number of trees they contain. The intensive farm has a plantation density of between two hundred and six hundred trees per hectare, while the super intensive farm has a plantation density of between one thousand and two thousand trees per hectare. Their olive trees are well aligned, meticulously maintained, and equally spaced within and between the rows.

At their plantations, Dominguez and Olivares grow two varieties of olives: Picual, a medium- to large-size olive that is very popular in Spain; and Arbequina, a smaller-size variety. Picual olives produce rich, green, pungent oil, while Arbequina olives render sweet oil. Dominguez and Olivares aim for intense green oil with notes rather similar to freshly cut grass, the tomato plant, or the Granny Smith apple.

In a real spirit of cooperation, these two farmers work closely together, especially at harvest time. Dominguez owns the mill, and Olivares has the know-how, providing all the technical knowledge for growing olives and producing premier oil. Growing olives and producing olive oil is their livelihood; they are proud of their brand of olive oil, Pago de Peñarrubia, which is also the name of Dominguez's mill.

Like many farmers to whom olive farming is a way of life in this vast olive oil production area of Castilla, these two fifth-generation olive farmers use a machine to pick olives from their 155 hectares of olive trees. Hand-picking is not an option here, as there are too many olives on the trees and, more importantly, processing must be done as soon as the olives are picked. The spacing of about 1.5 meters between the trees and careful pruning so the trees don't grow too tall are essential: the machine must be able to maneuver easily and not damage the trees.

Picking at the two orchards takes place in late October and into early November, when the olives are firm and mauve in color. Luckily for the pickers, the temperatures can drop to 25° C (77° F) in the fall.

Ten people work hard collecting the olives and getting them to the factory, while another ten work in the mill, cleaning, preparing, and processing the oil. With everyone working at top speed, they can pick and process the olives all in about six hours per day. The two owners provide accommodation for the hired hands as a way of making sure production is both continuous and efficient. As fermentation or oxidation starts the moment the fruit is picked, on certain days, they work much longer than six hours, managing to complete all of the harvesting and processing in two weeks.

Olivares and Dominguez use the modern centrifugal method and, in keeping with regulations to improve sustainability in Spain, use the two-way phase system. With so many olive oil producers in the country, waste treatment is hard to control with the three-way system.

The resulting oil is slightly cloudy because bits of sediment accumulate at the bottom of the container. There is some discussion amongst producers as to whether the oil should be filtered or not before bottling. Some prefer to keep the bits floating in the oil, which, according to the experts, contain more polyphenols. Others prefer to filter the oil, saying that the sediment eventually produces nondesirable flavors. Dominguez and Olivares prefer to filter the oil.

Olive By-Products

You might be surprised that to hear that when making olive oil, only 20 percent of the fruit is used. Other products are generated throughout the process, however—lesser-known products that we hardly think about. Some of these may even be considered valued by-products, crucial today for environmental and economic issues for the sector.

The month of March is a relatively slow time for European growers. This is the time to take a closer look at the trees in their orchards, making sure they are ready for the spring season. The vital task for them at this time is pruning the trees. If they want the best quality and quantity, they must remove the old branches; this stimulates and gives more strength to the buds. Olive branches can be utilized in many ways: they can be processed to make excellent cattle feed (instead of hay or straw) and can be used for making compost. Industrially, these excess branches are used for making paper, furniture, and fuel.

The by-products of processing oil are also beneficial and valuable. In some mills, extraction of oils starts in October and continues until February. The machines run continuously, producing oil as well as kilos of pomace and vegetable water. Pomace is a solid residue, a mixture of core, pulp, and skin. These two by-products can be treated on site, but in most cases, the pomace is bought by a dedicated processing company.

The pomace still contains a little olive oil, so to not lose a single drop, growers return the mixture for extracting at high temperatures, adding some solvents. This juice of the second press must not be confused with first cold pressing. The oil that comes out has no organoleptic qualities; it cannot be consumed in this state. This crude pomace oil will be sent to the refinery to be cleansed of all impurities and also to improve its smell, flavor, and color. Once "cleaned," it is added to extra-virgin olive oil and sold under the commercial category of olive pomace oil: edible but cheap. Olive pomace oil is also used in the manufacture of soap.

Today, the pomace and vegetable waters can be used in many ways. Pomace mixed with other components makes excellent fodder. The stone (pits) are used in boilers, and the pulp is made into fuel pellets for heating. The residue of vegetable water is a sensitive issue, as it is considered highly toxic to the environment. In Spain, for example, oil producers have to follow precise regulations for evacuating olive mill waste. Some producers, though, have discovered ways to use it as a garden fertilizer.

Studies on the antioxidation properties of some of the molecules contained in these by-products are now making news—scientists are looking closely at the fruit, olive pits, and leaves. The cosmetics industries see olive oil as a source of beauty, and new technologies are being developed to retrieve the phenolic compounds. One company even makes exfoliating sponges from olive pits.

Food trends are also changing. You can now find tea made from olive leaves in specialist boutiques, and surprisingly, in Japan, they make products like pasta made from ground olive leaves, soda from decanting the vegetable water, and fermented pomace to feed animals. At one university in Spain, they are currently looking into producing functional foods such as yogurt and drinks with enriched phenolic compounds.

Indeed, the business of the utilization of the humble olive is booming.

CONSUMPTION PER PERSON PER YEAR

GREECE
23 L

SPAIN
14 L

ITALY
12 L

FRANCE
2 L

United States consumption is less than 1L.

PART II

Here in Part II, we reveal the incredible discoveries of the seven wonders of olive oil. Each section focuses on uncovering the miraculous characteristics that we can use to improve our personal health by including olives and olive oil in our diets and lifestyles.

THE 7 WONDERS OF OLIVE OIL

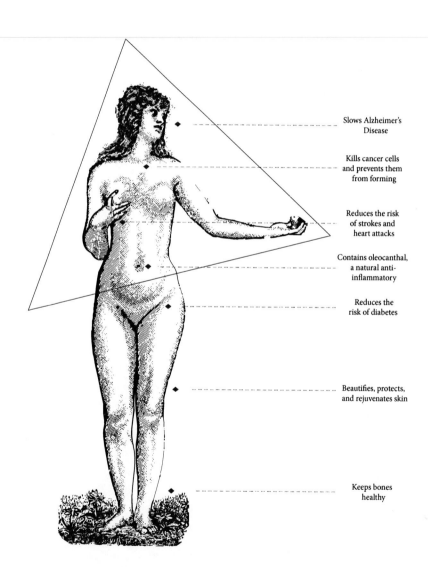

Slows Alzheimer's
Disease

Kills cancer cells
and prevents them
from forming

Reduces the risk
of strokes and
heart attacks

Contains oleocanthal,
a natural anti-
inflammatory

Reduces the
risk of diabetes

Beautifies, protects,
and rejuvenates skin

Keeps bones
healthy

OLIVE OIL CONTAINS OLEOCANTHAL, A NATURAL ANTI-INFLAMMATORY

Scientists discovered that extra-virgin olive oil contains oleocanthal, which mimics the activity of ibuprofen. Oleocanthal, like ibuprofen, may also be able to help reduce arthritis. Natural, safe extra-virgin olive oil can easily be incorporated into a daily diet, say researchers who have set up the Oleocanthal International Society.

When the American scientist Dr. Gary Beauchamp accepted an invitation to an olive oil symposium of newly pressed olive oil in Sicily, he had no idea it would change his life and the rest of the olive oil world. The sensory chemist was employed at the time at Monell Chemical Senses Center in Philadelphia, working specifically on a project relating to the medication ibuprofen. The anti-inflammatory drug stings as it goes down the throat; his job was to investigate why and to improve the taste.

Along with other scientists, food specialists, and chefs, he followed the precise and somewhat complicated instructions of how to taste olive oil. He cradled the cup, sipped, and slurped as he was told and promptly experienced a déjà vu moment: a burn in his throat, one that he recognized instantly as similar to liquid ibuprofen. The discovery in Italy was totally unexpected. Here were two unrelated compounds showing the same effects.

Delighted with his accidental scientific revelation, Dr. Beauchamp traveled back to Philadelphia, taking some of the precious oil with him. There, he and biologist Dr. Paul Breslin began investigating the properties of the pungent oil with their team. They isolated the throat-irritating compound, researched it, and named it "oleocanthal" from the Latin *oleo-*, olive, *canth-*, sting, and *-al*, aldehyde. They confirmed in further studies that although the chemical composition was different, the compound oleocanthal behaved similarly to the anti-inflammatory ibuprofen. (They discovered another miraculous wonder in oleocanthal, but we'll discuss that in the next chapter!)

Oleocanthal (OC) is a powerful antioxidant which develops when olives are crushed into pulp; this is what causes that sting, the peppery sensation in the back of the throat when you sip it neat. It comes from the purest of olive oil; if the oil stings a little, it contains only a little OC, but if it stings a lot, it contains a good amount of OC.

Interestingly, olive oil is the only vegetable oil that contains OC, that vital component with such pungency that it causes us to cough once or twice when we taste the green nectar. Some of us are more sensitive than others, but that distinct sting and irritation will vary depending on the variety of olives used to make the oil and also the concentration of extra-virgin olive oil.

Oleocanthal and Arthritis

So how does the ibuprofen-and-olive-oil connection help us?

Do you know anyone with rheumatoid arthritis? The word arthritis comes from the Latin word *itis*, which means "inflammation," and the Greek word *arthron*, meaning "joint." It is a chronic disease that can cause a great deal of pain. It starts off attacking the fingers and then the major joints, causing pain and stiffness in the mornings; it comes with fatigue, and, later on, it can cause permanent disability. Sadly, it gets worse with time unless the inflammation slows down.

Arthritis is quite simply inflammation of the joints caused by two inflammatory enzymes, COX-1 and COX-2. If the inflammation of these two enzymes continues unchecked, it causes damage to the cartilage and, eventually, the bones themselves. And once the deformity sets in, it cannot be reversed.

Doctors recommend anti-inflammatory drugs, in particular ibuprofen, to relieve pain and swelling from rheumatoid arthritis. Classed as a nonsteroidal anti-inflammatory drug (NSAID), ibuprofen helps reduce pain and inflammation, but unfortunately, it does not slow down the disease. Also important to remember is that long-term pain-relieving drugs are harmful to the body; even ibuprofen, taken over long periods, can cause damage to the kidneys as well as bring on intestinal bleeding.

Oleocanthal, like ibuprofen, inhibits production of the two enzymes that cause arthritis, but it does so without causing harm to the body. Scientists say oleocanthal is a natural anti-inflammatory compound, not structurally identical to ibuprofen but similar in potency and profile. Dr. Paul Breslin (who, you'll remember, helped Dr. Beauchamp with the initial studies) said that by inhibiting the two enzymes, inflammation and an increase in pain sensitivity becomes dampened. Now, the Arthritis Foundation recommends foods that are rich in antioxidants, like the Mediterranean diet, which emphasizes olive oil.

This is good news for sufferers of a disease that affects over two million people in the United States alone, most of them women. There is no cure yet for arthritis; sufferers can only follow treatment to reduce inflammation and pain and to prevent joint damage.

More tests are definitely needed, but wouldn't it be great if daily consumption of olive oil could help provide the same benefits of ibuprofen without the health risks? Dr. Beauchamp said that although we don't have enough evidence to tell us that eating olive oil daily can combat rheumatoid arthritis, eating a Mediterranean diet, with healthy amounts of olive oil and fats rich in omegas-3 and -6, appears to be beneficial.

Oleocanthal cannot totally replace drugs like ibuprofen, but consider it an herbal food—a natural remedy. And as you are looking for this natural remedy, remember that not all olive oils are the same; they don't all contain the same amount of oleocanthal, and there's nothing on the label to tell you how much or even if it contains any oleocanthal at all. To be sure you're getting the maximum oleocanthal, it's best to buy one from early-harvest olives or, in other words, newly pressed olive oil. When olives are picked green, they tend to have more polyphenols such as oleocanthal and are rich in antioxidants.

The University of California began to study how oleocanthal levels in olive oil varied and its impact on people. At a meeting held in Greece in October 2015, one of their research scientists, Dr. Roberta Holt, gave the results of the first clinical trials in humans using extra-virgin olive oil with a high concentration of oleocanthal and without it. Nine healthy male adults took part in the study where early-harvest Greek extra-virgin olive oil with high levels of oleocanthal and oleacein (another constituent of olive oil) was used.

Dr. Holt reported at the conference that the two compounds had a similar effect on the reactivity of blood platelets to a 400 milligram dose of ibuprofen.

As research continues, scientists are getting closer to understanding oleocanthal's protective role in our health while olive oil producers aim to get the maximum oleocanthal from their oil.

Oleocanthal could well be the most important polyphenol in olive oil; hopefully, it won't be long before the Oleocanthal Society publishes even more conclusive results based on human clinical studies.

The Oleocanthal International Society

The discovery of oleocanthal made such a buzz amongst researchers and health professionals that they formed a society. It started in June 2015 when retired Spanish physician José Antonio Amerigo, saddened to see that nothing had been done from 2005—when the compound was discovered—to 2013, decided to act. He contacted Gary Beauchamp and got the ball rolling.

The Oleocanthal International Society (OIS) was created.

The OIS today comprises scientists, nutritionists, physicians, dietitians, chefs, and even communication professionals, all from different countries and different backgrounds. Set up as a nonprofit group, the principal aim of the members is to facilitate and increase research into oleocanthal. Through collaboration and organized special events, members hope to publish their findings so as to promote and raise awareness of oleocanthal. The founding members met for the first time on the island of Zakynthos in Greece in early 2015. Dr. Breslin, also a founding member, said that as a biomedical researcher, he wanted to see research funding come from people who are interested in finding cures, preventions, and treatments for major killers like cancer, Alzheimer's disease, other terminal dementias, and diseases associated with chronic inflammation.

But it's not all research! The OIS also wants to help spread the word of the wonders of olive oil, for nutrition *and* flavor. For Dr. Amerigo and Chef Daniel García Peinado from Malaga in Spain, the interest is a mix of medicine and food. Dr. Amerigo wants to spread awareness of this natural food worldwide, while Peinado, at thirty-six, is a passionate, dynamic, health-conscious chef. Dr. Amerigo said it wasn't easy to find a young chef motivated by food cooked in extra-virgin olive oil but that Peinado was interested right in the beginning, that "rich oleocanthal was Peinado's guiding principle."

Dr. Amerigo added:

Cooking with olive oil for me means using it for grilling, in the oven, and even frying, because it enhances all dishes and is good for our health. Not so long ago, the University of Granada demonstrated how frying with olive oil increases the transfer of phenols from extra virgin to the vegetables. Soon, there will be other examples with meat, fish, etc.

These two OIS members now work in tandem, attending conferences, congresses, and cooking exhibitions to demonstrate how cooking with extra-virgin olive oil, rich in oleocanthal, is scientifically proven to be good for one's health.

Dr. Amerigo thinks we should be adding extra-virgin olive oil to our daily diet, about 40 milliliters (1.5 ounces) of oil, rich in oleocanthal, each day. He said, "65% of the Spanish olive groves are rich in oleocanthal." On a cautious note, though, he added, "We need to involve the producers as well because, although there's much olive oil being produced, we only get oleocanthal from extra-virgin olive oil."

In charge of gastronomy, Chef Daniel García Peinado is taking his work seriously and was voted second vice president of the group at the second OIS meeting in November 2015. Peinado says his primary role is to transmit and diffuse extra-virgin olive oil in the world of gastronomy, especially since the mix of gastronomy and medicine is a relatively new cooking concept. "Up until now," he said, "when we speak about healthy cuisine, we refer to diet therapy or calories but not based on anything as functional as EVOO, rich with oleocanthal, with scientifically proven health benefits."

Because of the OIS's efforts, we have made more discoveries about olive oil and greater awareness is being spread. Thank goodness that Dr. Beauchamp attended that olive oil symposium and noticed the first sign that olive oil contained a powerful anti-inflammatory element. Now we have several more wonders to discover!

OLIVE OIL FIGHTS AND PREVENTS CANCER

Studies have shown that olive oil has the ability to protect the body against certain benign and malignant tumors. In this chapter, we look at two common cancers: colon cancer and breast cancer.

You'll remember that Dr. Beauchamp and Dr. Breslin conducted the original discovery and research of oleocanthal. After recognizing the anti-inflammatory characteristics, Dr. Breslin continued investigating oleocanthal, this time looking at how and why cancer cells grow so quickly.

Focusing mainly on breast, pancreatic, and prostate cancer cells, Dr. Breslin headed a team of researchers as they applied oleocanthal to human cancer cells in the laboratory. The results were as unexpected as they were amazing! The team was surprised to see how quickly oleocanthal destroyed the cancer cells of the organs. The cells died within thirty to sixty minutes, unlike in other experiments and studies where cells programmed to die normally take between sixteen and twenty-four hours (scientists call this processed death "apoptosis"). Oleocanthal pierced the center of the cancer cell, targeting the lysosome, the part of the cell that stores waste. As it did so, it released the enzymes within the cell, causing it to die.

Dr. Breslin referred to the lysosome, which is full of aggressive enzymes, as "the garbage dump" of the cell. Lysosomes in cancer cells are larger than healthy cells, but what surprised the researchers was that oleocanthal did not damage the healthy cells in any way; it simply stopped their activity for a day. Dr. Breslin said, "It put the healthy cells to sleep for a day or so, then they resumed their activity. We now need to understand why cancerous cells are more sensitive to oleocanthal than noncancerous cells."

Could oleocanthal be the reason for reduced cancer incidence in the Mediterranean, where olive oil is consumed in high quantities?

When asked how much extra-virgin olive oil we should be consuming to reap the benefits of oleocanthal, Dr. Breslin said, "We need to separate OC from the plant and test it in toxicological studies to find out what [quantity] is safe. This has never been done, so we do not know how high a level would be tolerated well. In the meantime, I think 50 milliliters (2 ounces) of extra-virgin olive oil of a very high OC content each day appears both safe and desirable, provided people watch their total calorie intake."

The scientists say they still need a complete and thorough explanation of oleocanthal and to understand its protection mechanism in healthy cells. Once they achieve that, the next step will be to show that oleocanthal can shrink tumors in living animals.

Oleocanthal and Plasma Cells

Another study demonstrated the antitumor properties of oleocanthal, this time in a disease which affects blood plasma cells. This destructive cancer, called multiple myeloma (MM), involves the white blood cells made in the bone marrow, the soft center of the larger bones of our bodies. These plasma cells are vital because they are a part of our immune system; they produce antibodies which help fight infection. However, with MM, these abnormal cancer cells accumulate and push out the healthy blood cells.

Studies conducted in vitro have started to reveal the vast potential of the phenolic component of extra-virgin olive oil, mainly oleocanthal, in counteracting MM cell growth.

Spanish scientists from the NeuroEndocrine Interactions in Rheumatic and Inflammatory Diseases (NEIRID) laboratory described their results as "the first line of evidence that oleocanthal may be considered a novel antimyeloma drug, opening novel routes for the treatment of MM." How does olive oil do this? The group said that their experiments showed that oleocanthal eliminated the cancer cells by reducing the production of MIP-1 alpha, a key molecule which generates the myeloma cells.

Dr. Oreste Gualillo, head researcher, said, "This in vitro study suggests a therapeutic potential of oleocanthal in treating multiple myeloma."

Could oleocanthal work as a potential drug alone or with other established MM medicinal products for the treatment of MM in the future? When asked, Dr. Gualillo said, "Although the results are promising and suggest a wide spectrum of activity of certain molecules, further research on both in vitro and in vivo systems is always warranted."

So far, these anticancer properties of the compound were demonstrated in only in vitro studies; the real challenge will be, then, the follow-through with human trials. It may take a few years, but oleocanthal may well turn out to be effective anticancer treatment.

Extra-Virgin Olive Oil and Colon Cancer

Hydroxytyrosol, a component in olive oil, acts as a cancer suppressor in the intestine, protecting us from colon cancer. We should pay more attention to what we put on our plates because it eventually gets into our bowels.

Anne was speechless when the doctor told her she had bowel cancer; it came as a shock because the healthy, vivacious sixty-five-year-old had none of the listed factors that could affect her risk of colon cancer. Anne was not overweight, did not smoke, had no family members with the disease, nor was suffering from pain or discomfort. She was, however, sixty-five years old, an age at which the chances of developing colon cancer increase markedly. Anne had taken up the offer of a free stool test through a government screening program, but the report came back saying she had colon cancer. She was lucky; the doctors found her cancer in time, and even though she has to carry around a colonoscopy bag, she is responding well to treatment. Anne couldn't help but wonder: could she have avoided this disease by being more cautious with her food habits?

Today, this type of cancer is not considered life threatening, but people do not talk about it. There's nothing less glamorous than discussing changes in bowel habits and blood in the stool. Bowel cancer, also called colon cancer, is the second most common kind of cancer in the Western world. Doctors say it can be hereditary, or you can get it because of poor lifestyle habits and lack of exercise, but like hundreds of different cancers of the body, it occurs when cells of the affected area divide uncontrollably to form an abnormal mass.

In Anne's case, the disease was found in the last several inches of her colon as well as the rectum. As it started in the colon, the doctor said she had colon cancer. Sometimes, it can begin in the rectum, in which case it is diagnosed as rectal cancer, while cancers affecting either of these are called colorectal cancer. Unfortunately, the disease hardly shows any early signs and symptoms at the beginning stage and can progress long before it is detected, just as it did in Anne's case.

This is what happens to the body with colon cancer:

Colon cancer causes havoc with our endocannabinoid system—the body's central regulatory system—causing it to become unbalanced. You might not have heard of this complex process, a chemical messaging system discovered and identified only in the mid-1990s. It's not easy to explain how it all works, but what's important to know is that our bodies produce natural chemicals called endocannabinoids. These aren't stored in the body but are generated when necessary, binding to protein molecules or receptors present in cells throughout the body.

Endocannabinoids can change the way that a particular body part functions. Compare it to a lock-and-key system where the receptors are locks and cannabinoids act as keys: the two parts bind in a healthy system but are blocked in an unhealthy one.

With colon cancer, the intestinal receptors (known as CB1), although still present, get deactivated. However, CB1 is an anticancer agent recognized in the scientific world for its ability to suppress cancer growth.

Professor Mauro Maccorrone has been studying the cannabinoid's protective role. This is how he explains it:

> CB1 is like a guardian angel, a cancer suppressor. When the receptor is turned off, colorectal tumor growth starts. With this decrease in CB1, cancer-promoting cells become free to roam; they continue to grow and divide, eventually contaminating the surrounding tissues. Those cells lose the memory of how to die; they keep on growing.

Could olive oil have an effect on our endocannabinoid system? This was the question Maccorrone and his team set out to research: to understand and study the therapeutic properties of the phenols contained in extra-virgin olive oil and, more importantly, to see whether they had an anticancer effect by influencing the CB1 receptor.

Performing both in vitro and in vivo studies on human tissue and rats, the team carried out experiments using different grades of olive oil on colon cancer cells. They first discovered that high-quality extra-virgin olive oil contains hydroxytyrosol, the principal component able to protect the body from colon cancer.

According to Professor Maccorrone, "Hydroxytyrosol in extra-virgin olive oil wakes up the sentinels that allow our bodies to keep colorectal cancer away. The mixture of olive oil is essential, but it is the hydroxytyrosol that pulls the trigger." The researcher further explained that hydroxytyrosol activates the CB1 receptor through epigenetic mechanism. He continued to explain that with this genetic system, "extra-virgin olive oil doesn't break up or alter the genes; it just makes them more readable."

In the second part of their research study, the researchers fed rats a healthy diet with extra-virgin olive oil for ten days and then looked for changes in their cell linings. They found a significant increase in CB1 expression; extra-virgin olive oil had reactivated their CB1.

Maccorrone concluded from these experiments that adding olive oil to an animal's diet can restore a healthy CB1 receptor level to protect cells against cancer; in other words, high-quality olive oil can defend us against colorectal cancer!

Consider colorectal cancer a food-related cancer, then think of the amount of food we ingest in a lifetime. Diet is bound to have a direct impact on colorectal cancer, because everything we eat passes through the digestive system, into the intestine, and out of the rectum. But food is customer oriented these days, where we, the consumers, often ignore the food value chain, not bothering to learn much about where the food came from and what processes were involved before it got to our plate.

Keeping the entire intestinal system healthy and manageable is important to allow the body to convert food into energy and get rid of waste. Adding olive oil to the daily diet can help with elimination and regulation by lubricating the whole system. It allows the food we ingest to have a smooth passage right through the digestive track, softening the stools in the rectum and making them easier to pass. It also works as a mild laxative, so if we use olive oil regularly, we should not be constipated. Choosing a higher quality of olive oil is crucial. A better-quality olive oil has more flavors and is much more efficient.

An interesting animal test showed promising results in the fight against colon cancer. In Barcelona, researchers wanted to see how olive oil compared with other oils, to study the effects of olive oil on the colon. The scientists fed mice with diets rich either in safflower oil, fish oil, or olive oil. The oils were mixed with a chemical to accelerate cancer in the bowel and given to half of the three groups. The study lasted five months, after which the doctors at the University Hospital Clinic of Barcelona Department of Gastroenterology noted that twice as many rats in the safflower group developed colon cancer as in the two other groups. What's interesting here is that these oils have different chemical structures: olive oil is a monounsaturated fat, a good type of fat, which significantly reduced the number of cancer lesions. The medical professionals said that the benefits could have been due to a lowering of inflammatory chemicals in the intestine.

Today, we have a mass of information at our disposal, knowledge passed on from clinicians and nutritionists telling us the importance of eating the right food. However, the statistics are still high: the Center for Disease Control and Prevention (CDC) reports that colorectal cancer is the third most common cancer and the second leading cause of cancer-related deaths in the United States. Instead of reaching for a drug to "treat" a digestive symptom, we should perhaps choose more carefully what we put into our mouths.

As Professor Maccorrone pointed out, we seem to forget the "importance of the quality of food, and that includes olive oil." The Italian specialist in Food Science and Human Nutrition thinks that more could be done by food manufacturers to show the authenticity of their products through correct labeling. Consumers can easily be seduced by the impressive *Made in Italy* label, but, as he says, the label might say *Italian Olive Oil* when the olives come from somewhere else entirely. Professor Maccorrone feels food awareness could start at school and that lawmakers should work harder at defending quality, adding that "we all know this is happening, but there's not enough reaction against it. I would like to see more healthy food and a deeper respect for genuine, natural food."

The hard truth, however, is that poor-quality oil and deception in the olive oil business is not new. Extra-virgin olive oil is very often in the spotlight when it comes to food fraud, and even some of the best-known brands and most highly reputed companies have been caught trying to pass off a virgin oil or simply olive oil as "extra-virgin" when it is not truly the same quality. With olive oil fraud, industrialists take advantage of the consumer's ignorance and a lack of controlled chemical and sensory tests to mix extra virgin with another vegetable oil such as rapeseed oil (also known as colza). Sadly, this widespread, deceitful, and damaging practice is likely to continue until food authorities enforce stricter laws. As consumers, we need to remember that high-quality olive oil is better for us and that fraudulent oil does not offer the same health benefits as extra-virgin olive oil.

One thing is clear in the fight against colon cancer: good food is a lot kinder to our body than drugs, especially extra-virgin olive oil, which is shown to help take care of our bowels.

Olive Oil Works Effectively to Fight Breast Cancer

It is very hard for women to live with breast cancer. Studies show that women who follow a Mediterranean diet can reduce their risks of getting the disease. Various components in olive oil help lower the risks of breast cancer.

Slim, attractive, forty-year-old Joanna answered with a smile when she heard her name called; it was her turn to go to the X-ray room. She had come for her yearly checkup at the busy Symptomatic Breast Clinic. Breast technologists have learned how to be discreet in their work; they know how vital it is to be sensitive to the anxiety of their patients when they come for their follow-up mammogram. It was not easy, though, to be discreet with Joanna. As she took her shirt off, you had to look, admire, and take in the stunning work of art running up the right side of her chest. Starting from her slim waist and going up to where her breast should have been was a truly magnificent tattoo: a rose shrub with vibrant green leaves, ending at the top with a magnificent pink rose. It replaced the breast Joanna once had.

She explained, "Trees are a symbol of life; this tattoo is sacred to me. After my mastectomy, I needed something to remind me that life must go on. This tattoo is what helps me not to be fearful of the future."

The young patient had been diagnosed with breast cancer three years before. No one in her family had had breast cancer, yet she could not ignore the lump in her breast; it seemed to be getting bigger every day. She eventually saw her general practitioner, who referred her to a diagnostic breast unit. She then had to see a surgeon.

After she'd had the tests, the surgeon gave her the bad news. He told her, "You have a choice: you can have either a mastectomy or a wide local excision." Then he explained the difference. A mastectomy would remove her entire breast; a wide local excision would remove the cancer and some of the normal tissue around it, "but the cancer could come back," he warned.

Joanna explained why she made the decision to have a mastectomy. "The choice sounded drastic at the time, but I did not want to leave any doubts. I could not afford to. I had to think of my family; the kids were still young." Shockingly early to be diagnosed with an aggressive form of breast cancer, Joanna admits she had to face many challenges—the most important, she confesses, was fear.

Women with breast cancer who are being treated, even those that have successfully been treated, all say the same thing—they are always haunted by fear and trepidation. They fear that the cancer will come back. The medical term for this is a "recurrence," and it can happen five, ten, or even fifteen years after the necessary therapy. The treatment itself to remove or destroy the cancer is stressful whether it is done through surgery, chemotherapy, or radiation therapy; they all leave changes to the body, as well as visible scars that make women feel uncomfortable with themselves.

There's no one single reason women get breast cancer, but it seems that several factors can contribute: genes, lifestyle, environment, and hormones are the chief risk factors, and any combination can trigger the disease.

Women over fifty are more likely to have breast cancer; that is why some countries have a breast cancer program for older women. These screening programs allow women to have mammograms—breast X-rays—either every two or three years (depending on the country) as well as free health treatment if they are diagnosed with the disease.

Some women can inherit abnormal genes, which means that their risk of developing breast cancer is much higher than someone who does not have those genes. The actress Angelina Jolie made the decision to have preventive double mastectomy surgery when she realized she carried the same genes as her deceased mother.

Cancer of the breast starts when cells begin to grow in an uncontrolled way, forming a tumor. The cancer is noninvasive if the cancer cells are only in the breast and have not spread any further. However, when cancer spreads and invades the surrounding tissue, it is called invasive breast cancer. Most invasive cancers spread to the rest of the body if they are not treated in time. They pass through the bloodstream and lymphatic system, forming secondary cancers in other parts of the body.

Joanna lives in the UK, where cancer rates are high. According to Cancer Research UK, there were 53,700 new cases of invasive breast cancer in 2013, and it was the most common cause of cancer death that year. A breast screening program in the UK provides a free service, aiming to find breast cancers early in women. A recent extension now includes women aged between forty-seven and seventy-three. It means that women who are registered with their local general practitioners receive letters of invitation every three years to attend a dedicated screening unit for a routine mammogram. If the results appear abnormal, they are then asked to participate in an assessment clinic where they might have new images, ultrasounds, and perhaps a biopsy. Breast Screening UK says that one in every twenty-five women who are called back for assessment is diagnosed with breast cancer.

The Mediterranean Diet Lowers the Risk

As women get older, their risk of getting breast cancer increases. They also have to put up with menopause, which has a definite influence on breast cancer. And life expectancies in Western countries are also increasing. This means that the proportion of women affected by breast cancer is continually growing.

The results of the following study are significant because it focuses specifically on postmenopausal women, where the need for prevention and control is more vital these days.

The data in this study was the first randomized trial to research whether a Mediterranean diet could protect women from breast cancer. It was a parallel study carried out in conjunction with studies on cardiovascular disease by PREDIMED (Prevención con Dieta Mediterránea). PREDIMED researchers were primarily concerned with nutrition and heart disease, but the trial was also designed to follow the incidence of five different types of cancer, including breast cancer in older women.

Researchers chose older subjects for this study, Spanish women between the ages of sixty and eighty, who were almost all menopausal. None of them had cardiovascular disease, but all had either type 2 diabetes or at least three of the major cardiovascular risk factors that could bring on the disease; these included smoking, hypertension, or family history of cardiovascular diseases. They all had an average body mass index of 30; in other words, they were obese. This in itself is a known risk for breast cancer.

The researchers divided the 4,282 women into three groups:

- 1,476 were put on a Mediterranean diet supplemented with extra-virgin olive oil. All the women were given a liter of olive oil every week to make sure they followed the specification required by the research team. These Spanish women use the oil anyway; it is what they are used to using, as Spain is the largest producer of olive oil.

- 1,285 were instructed to follow the Mediterranean diet supplemented with a daily intake of 30 grams of mixed nuts. They received weekly supplies of nuts during the research period.

- 1,392 received dietary training and were asked to follow a low-fat diet.

After a follow-up period of about five years, the researchers found that thirty-five women had developed malignant breast cancer. The results revealed that the women who followed the Mediterranean diet supplemented with olive oil showed a 68% lower risk than those who were on the control diet. Those in the second group with nut supplements showed a 40% lower risk of breast cancer than the control group.

The researchers concluded that preventive strategies represented the most sensible approach to treating cancer. They said they hoped to see more emphasis on a Mediterranean diet to reduce cancer and cardiovascular disease and improve overall health and well-being. They recognized, however, that the results could be considered limiting because all the participants were from Spain, were white, and lived where the Mediterranean diet and cooking with olive oil is a way of life. We have to remember that the Spanish volunteers already consumed significantly less saturated fats than Americans, Canadians, and the British.

Another limiting factor is that this was a secondary analysis, carried out in conjunction with the study of cardiovascular disease. It was concerned primarily with women with a high cardiovascular risk rather than a risk for breast cancer. What it does show, however, is that prevention of breast cancer might very well start in our kitchens.

The following large-scale studies also show the importance of consuming the right type of food.

The Mediterranean Diet and Greek Women

A poor and high-fat diet seems to be one of the leading causes of breast cancer, which is much more prevalent in Western countries. The Mediterranean diet, on the other hand, is rich in antioxidants and contains only a small amount of animal saturated fats. This study looks specifically at the association of breast cancer and the Mediterranean diet in a Mediterranean country.

14,807 women took part in the European Prospective Investigation into Cancer and Nutrition (EPIC), and the results were published in the highly regarded *American Journal of Clinical Nutrition.*

This study looked at what the women ate; it followed their eating habits for nearly ten years. The Greek women started the research by answering an in-depth questionnaire about their diet to see how they conformed to the Mediterranean diet. From that, they were given a score from 1 to 9. Those who adhered to typical dietary components got the high score of 9, while those with minimum adherence scored 1.

At the end of the study, 240 cases of breast cancer were reported. In their report, the researchers indicated that, in premenopausal women, there was "no significant association between conformity to the diet and breast cancer risk." What they did find, though, was an inverse situation with postmenopausal women. They concluded that "conformity to the traditional Mediterranean diet is associated with a lower risk of breast cancer amongst postmenopausal women." The report added that this could explain the lower incidence of breast cancer in Mediterranean countries.

Prevention Is a Better Cure

The Genesis Breast Cancer Prevention Centre in the United Kingdom understands how important it is to tackle breast cancer and to prevent breast cancer from developing. This UK charity is dedicated entirely to the prediction and prevention of breast cancer. The team believes that if women understand the factors that cause breast cancer, they will take positive steps to lower their risk and prevent the disease.

One of those factors is maintaining a healthy lifestyle. Studies show that an unhealthy lifestyle increases the risk of breast cancer; carrying excess weight, being sedentary, and consuming high amounts of alcohol are all strongly associated with breast cancer. To put it bluntly, we eat the wrong food, and too much, and don't exercise enough; this is why we carry that excess weight and increase our risk.

At Genesis, they developed an efficient eating plan for women at increased risk of breast cancer who are overweight, want to lose weight, and, once that is achieved, want to maintain a healthy weight to reduce their risk. Michelle Harvie is the only UK dietician who has performed in-depth studies on the relationship between diet and breast cancer prevention. Based on these research studies and trials at Genesis, she has developed a two-day diet approach to how we can reduce our calorie intake and have less sugar and processed food.

A daily diet can be restrictive, too hard to follow for many people, but with this eating plan, dieters do not check their calorie intake or skip meals; "they simply follow a low-carb plan for two days and eat sensibly for the rest of the week."

Dr. Harvie says: "We advise our patients to try to follow our two-day diet, which includes the benefits of two days of energy restriction and five days of a healthy Mediterranean diet." Dr. Harvie recommends a healthy diet such as the Mediterranean diet— which includes fish, fruit, vegetables, low-fat dairy, high-fiber carbohydrates, and moderate amounts of healthy fats like olive oil and nuts—for women who wish to reduce their risk of breast cancer and other diseases. She feels that this diet increases satiety and prevents overeating, which are key to reducing weight.

Studies show that incidences of breast cancer decrease with an increased intake of olive oil, highly present in the Mediterranean diet, but you may ask: what components in olive oil actually help lower the incidence of breast cancer?

Dr. José Gafario from the University of Jaén in Spain has been studying the effects of some of the minor components in olive oil, looking at compounds which could play a natural role in preventing disease. The research team carried out in vitro studies on squalene, one of the oil's minor polyphenols with strong antioxidant properties on healthy human breast tissue and cancerous human cells. You may not have heard of squalene, but squalene got its name because it is derived from shark liver oil. Although present in other edible oils, the concentration in olive oil is much higher, ranging from between 0.8 to 13 grams per kilogram, depending on the olive variety.

Dr. Gafario reported that "squalene protects the DNA of healthy mammary epithelial cells against oxidative damage, suggesting that this molecule could have the potential to prevent human breast cancer." He said that squalene appeared to have a preventive role in the healthy cells but less potential in tumor cells.

The team also studied the effect of oleanolic acid, another compound found in the olive skin and leaves of the olive tree. These tests were also carried out on healthy breast cells as well as cancerous ones. Dr. Gafario said that the results suggested a dual effect on healthy and tumor cells and that the data from the studies suggested that "oleanolic acid could be a chemo preventive agent" (a food or drug that prevents or delays cancer) in human breast cancer. He added that, at the same time, it "could have the ability to inhibit proliferation of highly invasive breast cancer cells."

In normal breast cells, on the other hand, the effects of oleanolic acid were different. He said that in normal breast cells, the effect is the opposite: it appears to decrease oxidative stress (which we'll discuss further later) and protects the DNA (our genes) against oxidative damage. A reduction of oxidation stress is good news! Our bodies are in danger of too much oxidation stress, the medical term used when our cells are not protected adequately from potential damage, perhaps because of a lack of antioxidant nutrients. Not enough antioxidant nutrients suggest that eating habits are not what they should be.

Interestingly, other scientific researchers have described other positive effects of oleanolic acid against other diseases; the effects of oleanolic acid are certainly not limited to breast cells.

There is one other element of olive oil that needs to be addressed in how it can fight or prevent cancer. Olive oil contains vitamin E. Though we will discuss it further later, it is important to recognize that vitamin E is an antioxidant that protects our cells from damage. The chemical name is "tocopherol," and olive oil is rich in vitamin E (alpha-tocopherol).

How does vitamin E work for us? Because it is a powerful antioxidant, it neutralizes the free radicals—the unstable molecules of oxygen that cause havoc to our DNA and eventually cause cancer. Vitamin E is often described as the scavenger of free radicals. Research shows that the best form of the vitamin is what we get from our food supply naturally, as our bodies do not absorb the artificial form as well.

Is It Just a Question of Fats?

A study which took place in Sweden differs from the above Mediterranean research because it did not take place in the Mediterranean area and also looked specifically at the intake of fats. The report came from the Karolinska Institutet in Stockholm; it was a major study involving 61,000 women, all between the ages of forty and seventy and born between 1914 and 1948.

The women filled in questionnaires that listed sixty-seven common foods, with further, more specific questions about the participants' fat consumption. The researchers then checked the Cancer Registry to see who in the group developed breast cancer. Between 1987 and 1993, there were 674 confirmed cases of invasive breast cancer. When researchers analyzed the data, they found that a high intake of monounsaturated fats—the fat you get from olive oil—was protective against breast cancer. They found that a high intake of polyunsaturated fats raised the risk of developing breast cancer considerably, reporting that a 5-gram increment in the daily intake of polyunsaturated fats corresponded to a 69% increase in risk. The researchers said that monounsaturated fat in the diet appeared to reduce the likelihood of breast cancer by 45%. It appeared that saturated fat—the kind found in meat and dairy products—had no effect on breast cancer one way or the other.

Interestingly, they found that the largest contributor to polyunsaturated fats came from margarine (33%), followed by bread and cereals (23%), meat (17%), and dairy products (11%).

These study results show the importance of the kinds of fats we eat. Eating the wrong fats can be dangerous.

Olive Oil versus Corn Oil

Studies have shown that we have such a high rate of breast cancer because of the kind of fat we eat. Trans fats, the sort of fat we get from packaged fats, is particularly dangerous for our health. Scientists compared the effect of different oils on rats, looking at corn oil—a source of omega-6 acids and considered a polyunsaturated fat—and olive oil, a monounsaturated fat. The two groups of rats were fed with the two oils, while the control group was given a low-fat diet. They injected rats with powerful doses of carcinogens and looked at the resulting development of breast cancer in the two groups. They found that the rats fed with corn oil developed more numerous breast cancers more quickly than those on the olive oil diet. These rats also developed more body weight. Those on olive oil, however, did not show any increase in body weight, and they showed fewer tumors, which developed much more slowly than those on the corn oil.

How do the researchers explain the result?

They say that a diet high in corn oil stimulates certain proteins that allow the cancer cells to grow uncontrollably. The diet based on olive oil, on the other hand, reduces the activity of these proteins and encourages cell destruction.

In the fight against breast cancer, there are factors such as genetics and age that we cannot control. We do have a choice, though, when it comes to lifestyle and diet. A good healthy intake of olive oil is one of those healthy choices that can make a difference.

What Oil You Should Be Using and When: A guide to choosing the right cooking oil

Which cooking oil should you be using?

All oils are not created equally; they come with different health benefits and nutrition. One thing is clear: vegetable oils enhance the taste of foods and dishes. Besides being tasty, they are necessary for our balance because they are essential to the body and ensure proper functioning of our cells. Vegetable oils have the advantage of not containing cholesterol, unlike animal fats such as butter. Some vegetable oils are essential because our bodies do not produce certain elements in them, so we need to get them from our diet. Omega-3 and -6 acids are good examples.

As oils do not all have the same composition, even though they have the same caloric value of 9 kilocalories, it is best to mix and choose them according to the specific type of cooking.

"No oil is perfect, so it is best to choose carefully, and don't hesitate to mix them," says Silvie Borrat, who is a pharmaceutical assistant and phyto-aromatherapist in Toulouse, France. "For the healthy functioning of our body, it is important to consume fat. It is recommended to reduce the intake of animal fats and to promote the intake of vegetable lipids. Each vegetable oil is made, in varying proportions, of saturated fatty acids, monounsaturated oils, or polyunsaturated oils. Mixing them gives a complete diet in different compounds for good health," she explains. To fully benefit from their contents and to create good balance, it is important to alternate, mix, and vary their use. The change also means developing the palate to appreciate new flavors; it is essential to use them reasonably to enjoy the benefits of each.

Remember: not only the brain but also the retina, skin, and bones need essential fatty acids for growth. Oils also help maintain general good health throughout our lifetime. We should choose cold-pressed oils and organic oils if possible.

Here's what you need to know:

- We need fats to be healthy.
- The healthiest oils must be cold pressed and organic.
- Oils rich in omega-3s cannot stand the heat and are, therefore, best used cold.
- We should limit our intake of omega-6 unsaturated fatty acids, which promote inflammation.
- Try mixing different oils. A good example of this is vinaigrette made with olive oil and linseed oil. This mixture allows you to have both omega-3s and -9s.

⇴ To conserve our health and to safeguard our planet, we should avoid soybean oil and palm oil.

OLIVE OIL

Olive oil contains more than 60% of monounsaturated fats, omega-9s, a few omega-6s, and vitamin E. Olive oil is an essential oil in the kitchen; there is nothing better for cooking vegetables. Olive oil can easily replace butter or sunflower oils in cooking. For salad dressings, mix olive oil with a little linseed oil or walnut oil to get that healthy omega-3 content.

PEANUT OIL

Peanut oil, also called groundnut oil, is high in omega-6 (34%) and omega-9 (48%) acids. It has no omega-3s. This means it tolerates heat well. Peanut oil is a good choice for frying.

Be careful, though: allergy to peanuts is a very common sensitivity.

COLZA OIL OR RAPESEED OIL

Colza oil, rapeseed oil, or canola oil (in Canada and America) contains omega-9 (57%), omega-6 (23%), and omega-3 (10–15%) acids. It is the newest oil on the market, but scientists disagree about the effects it can have on our health. As over 90% of canola oil is genetically modified, processing of this oil can be a real concern.

NUT OIL

Nut oil has a perfect ratio of omega-6 and omega-3 acids. Its biggest asset is its superb taste. Nut oil cannot stand the heat, though, so keep it away from all heat and oven use.

COCONUT OIL

Coconut oil is rich in saturated fatty acids; recent studies show that it is not as bad for health as the saturated acids we get from animals. It contains medium-chain fatty acids that provide a quick source of energy and could even have positive health benefits. More studies are being carried out, but one thing is sure: coconut oil is becoming more and more popular in cosmetics. The smoke point is high.

SUNFLOWER OIL, GRAPESEED OIL, AND CORN OIL

These oils contain more than 50% of omega-6 unsaturated fatty acids that can increase inflammation in the body. We should limit their consumption in our diet or mix them with other oils with a large number of omega-3s.

Sunflower oil, with a high content of oleic acid, is produced from hybrid plants. It has a composition similar to olive oil and is also more stable than traditional varieties. However, it is hard to find these oils cold pressed.

SOYBEAN OIL

The composition of soybean oil is not great for our health, as it contains little omega-9 and omega-3 acids but more than 50% of omega-6 acids. We should consume soybean oil only occasionally and ensure that we buy organic.

PALM OIL

The attractive price and excellent heat resistance of palm oil make it the preferred industrial oil. It contains 50% saturated fatty acids and little omega-3 acids, not a very good composition for our health. Also, it poses a problem for the planet when not grown from sustainable palm groves. In contrast, red palm oil (available at health food stores) contains vitamin E and carotene and can replace butter.

Linseed oil or flaxseed oil

This oil is perfect for vegetarians because it contains more than 50% omega-3s. With an extremely high rate of omega-3s, flaxseed oil rectifies the imbalance between omega-6 and omega-3 acids that prevails today in the United States.

Because it is so rich in omega-3s, you cannot use it for cooking, so it can only be used in vinaigrettes. It hasn't got a very pleasant taste, so it is a good idea to mix it with tastier oil. The ideal pairing is one part linseed oil and two parts olive oil to mask the taste. To avoid the problem of the oil going bad, linseed oil should be refrigerated. Flaxseed oil is found only in health food stores and can be a little expensive.

Cod liver oil

Cod liver oil is very rich in omega-3s and efficient on the cardiovascular system. It also makes our cell membranes more fluid and boosts our morale. Cod liver oil contains vitamin D, essential for growth, and high levels of vitamin A, which is great for fighting infection. However, it has an especially bad taste. It is better to take it in capsules or eat cod liver on toast.

Other oils

Argan oil, borage oil, and sweet almond oil are very popular in cosmetics.

COMPOSITION OF FATTY ACID
OF THE MAIN VEGETABLES OILS

DIETARY FATS   FATTY ACID CONTENT NORMALIZED TO 100 PERCENT

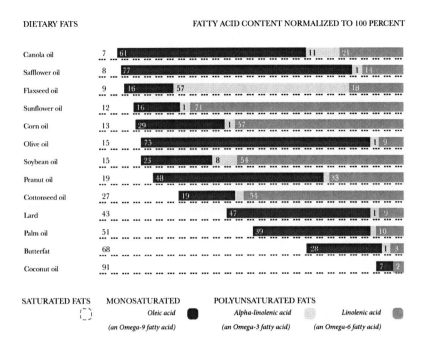

	Canola oil	7	61		11	21
Safflower oil	8	77		1	14
Flaxseed oil	9	16	57		18
Sunflower oil	12	16	1	71
Corn oil	13	29	1	57
Olive oil	15	75		1	9
Soybean oil	15	23	8	54
Peanut oil	19	48		33
Cottonseed oil	27	19	54
Lard	43	47		1	9
Palm oil	51	39		10
Butterfat	68	28	1	3
Coconut oil	91	7	2

SATURATED FATS   MONOSATURATED   POLYUNSATURATED FATS
                  Oleic acid ⬤   *Alpha-linolenic acid*   *Linolenic acid* ⬤
                  (an Omega-9 fatty acid)   *(an Omega-3 fatty acid)*   *(an Omega-6 fatty acid)*

OLIVE OIL BEAUTIFIES, PROTECTS, AND REJUVENATES SKIN

For centuries, olive oil has been recognized as an amazing substance, a beautiful gift with many uses. We now know more about the different ingredients that work toward healthier skin: vitamin E, vitamin K, phenols, and squalene. Although they weren't aware of the scientific knowledge we have today, the Greeks were among the first to cultivate, appreciate, and use olive oil extensively.

At the first Olympic Games in 776 BC, winners received olive tree branches cut with a gold-handled knife—an offering of peace. But the ancient Greeks also used olive oil in cosmetics. They loved beauty, considering it a blessing and a gift from the gods. At the Olympic Games, wrestlers used to rub olive oil on their skins before entering the arena. Just imagine how their torsos must have shone in the strong Mediterranean sunshine. They were probably not very comfortable, but to the crowds who came to watch them, they appeared strong, sturdy, and beautiful. The contestants believed that by anointing themselves with the oil, the goddess Athena would bestow power, strength, and wisdom as they fought. Rubbing olive oil on their body during training was standard practice at the time—it protected their bodies, elasticizing and soothing their muscles at the same time.

Later on, the Greeks and the Romans discovered the pleasures of bathhouses—a place to wash, chat, and contemplate. They would spend hours in these baths, enjoying the custom of anointing their bodies with olive oil, rubbing it well into the skin then scraping away all the accumulated dirt and sweat. They used a bronze metal tool for this oil cleansing, a kind of spatula called a strigil with a curved blade at the end which made it look dangerous; but it was just thick enough to skim the surface without cutting the skin. This was the first known exfoliating tool, used in what we can describe as the equivalent of our modern-day spa.

Olive oil became more and more popular as the people discovered its health and beauty benefits. Surprising as it may seem, the discovery of soap came well after exfoliants. The origin of soap is not quite clear, but we know that the first documented olive soaps (created in Marseille around 1370) were made using simple products combined with seawater and local olive oil. Increasing demands for Savon de Marseille at the beginning of the seventeenth century lead to overworked employees in the many factories, which in turn caused the quality of the soap to deteriorate.

Factories were springing up everywhere at the time, with production figures reaching as high as twenty thousand tons per year in France. A French law passed in 1668 changed that. The new regulations limited the use of the name "Savon de Marseille" to soaps made only in and around Marseille. It stipulated that only pure olive oil should be used, that no fat could be added, and that certain manufacturing processes had to be respected; only then could the soap carry the prestigious Marseille mark.

Today, Marseille is still the principal place for producing Savon de Marseille soap, with around ten savonnières (soap factories) in and around the city. Although production methods and contents have changed over time, many French people still recognize the olive oil–based soap as a traditional soap, one that their mothers and grandmothers used. For many, it is a simple, pure, natural, and hypoallergenic soap, ideal for people with sensitive skin.

Portrait of an Olive Oil Soap Maker

Nia Hafsia and her husband, Karim, live in a tiny village called Bourgnac, a beautiful little village with only 350 inhabitants situated in southwest France between Bordeaux and Bergerac. Their property, an old flour mill, dates from 1657 and comprises a thousand square meters where they have their home, Nia's soap workshop, and a boutique all on the same premises.

Indeed, this is the inspirational and motivating environment of artists and creators. This is where Nia lives her passion—making olive oil–based soaps, lotions, and creams. A true artist, she uses natural plant colors and clays in her soaps, ingeniously swirling and marbling the eight-kilo blocks of soap to transform them into true works of art. Her other specialty, she says, is blending the natural essential oils and absolutes (concentrated oil mixtures from plants). Mixing different natural perfumes together not only creates beautiful fragrances that smell good but also yields positive, therapeutic benefits for various skin types.

Her beautiful olive oil soaps are mild and gentle, cleansing without drying the skin. The secret is in the blending of natural fatty acids that help protect and regenerate the skin, leaving it soft and smooth. She uses between 50% and 80% extra-virgin olive oil in her base formula. Because of the quality oil, Nia said that individuals with sensitive skin can use her products, as the soap has soothing and nourishing properties.

Nia launched her natural, handmade soap–making business, Passion Savon, some thirty-five years ago in Wales in the United Kingdom. The venture started in her kitchen, where she could work and stay at home with her four young children. Today, the small cottage industry has snowballed into a business that manufactures one ton of soap every two months. Nia researches, blends, refines, and creates her products, increasing production to satisfy customers not only in France but also in China, Hong Kong, Lebanon, Dubai, Sweden, Holland, Malta, Finland, the United States, South Africa, and many other countries throughout the world.

As a qualified aromatherapist, she recognizes how important it is to protect and preserve the skin—the largest organ of the body—without compromising our environment. For her organic soap products, she uses only 100% natural raw ingredients, many of which are sourced locally from small producers. She says the great thing about olive oil is that it does not block the pores and that it makes soap that is suitable even for babies, children, and elderly people with fragile skin types. The extra-virgin olive oil that she uses is first cold pressed and food quality.

She explains, "A lot of soap manufacturers add palm oil to the soap mixture, but palm oil is a saturated fat, which can be damaging to the health and also to the environment, as its production is threatening our rainforests." Nia's company has a strict no–palm oil policy. "We feel that the product is destroying our rainforests, and many animals are losing their habitats because of the intensive industry that is slashing and burning trees, leaving a barren wasteland where there was once life."

Many soap makers choose a cheaper option for their craft, using the less expensive pomace oil, the last grade of olive oil. These are dregs that are that are washed with a chemical solvent. Nia feels that it should not even be referred to as "olive oil."

Passion Savon uses a true cold process saponification (the natural chemical process of soap making) for manufacturing their soap. And Nia mixes her soap at an ambient temperature of between 20° C and 24° C (68° F and 75° F). "It's like cooking vegetables. If we overcook them, all the precious nutrients are lost. We don't heat the ingredients included in our soap formula, thereby preserving the positive therapeutic properties in the final soap bar."

The company does not just make healthy, olive oil–based products; they are also very aware of the duty that small enterprises have to protect the environment. They manufacture solid products that do not need packaging. Nia says, "I hate the thought of those millions and zillions of plastic bottles that are cluttering, polluting, and ruining our world." At Passion Savon, they pack their skincare range, Kariti, in special dark glass containers, without water content, so there is no need for chemical preservatives, and the twelve products are concentrated and based on organic, effective, and active raw materials.

Nia says that adding olive oil to cosmetics and beauty products gives the skin wonderful moisturizing properties in the same way as the soap, but in a more profound way, because soap is a "wash off" product whereas creams and lotions are "leave on" products. Without giving any secrets away, she says that a very simple and easy moisturizing cream can be made with 30% extra-virgin olive oil, 5% vegetable emulsifying wax, 5% shea butter, 5% vegetable glycerin, and 55% rose water or aloe vera.

Even though the price of extra-virgin olive oil has increased tremendously, Nia makes no compromise in her choice of natural, high-quality, organic, and free-trade ingredients. She would not dream of changing anything and is determined to keep using this top-grade oil for her luxury, artisanal soaps. This is good news when you consider that today the market is full of detergent-based liquid and solid soaps, shower gels, shampoos, and bubble baths, mostly formulated with a base of sodium lauryl sulphate, sodium laureth sulphate, or ammonium laureth sulphate, all harsh chemicals that can be dangerous for our health.

Nia's spirit of innovation, environmental awareness, talent, and hard work have not gone unnoticed. In January 2016, she received the outstanding award of Maître Artisan d'Art in recognition for her work as an aromatherapist and master soap maker. Translated as "master of art," this is France's prestigious award, honoring her as one of a selection of the country's most gifted master artisans. She deserves this recognition for her hard work and is the first Welsh woman to receive this diploma in her field of work. The mayor of her village, Bourgnac, was there to support her, pleased to put their village "on the map," so to speak. Nia enthuses, "It means that I am recognized as a specialist and master of art in my work, and that is really thrilling."

The company is busy developing the business further to include more exciting, original, and innovative aromatherapy olive oil products. The vivacious entrepreneur says excitedly, "The future looks bright! The company continues to grow, and my creative skills seem to grow with it. I am so grateful to be able to live in such a beautiful and safe part of the world and be able also to have a job that is such a real pleasure. It's incredible to wake up each morning and be excited to go over to my workshop and see my new 'babies' that I made the day before."

Squalene and Squalane in Cosmetics

Squalene is a natural compound present in the outer layer of our skin, making up roughly 10% of our serum; it is a lipid that protects us from environmental toxins and helps to retain moisture. The richest source that people have cultivated, however, comes from sharks, followed by extra-virgin olive oil. Our natural squalene contributes to hydrating the body, but after age thirty or so, the body levels start declining, and by age fifty, the production levels drop. Squalene has another downside: it is highly unstable and so cannot be used in cosmetics or skincare products that need a long shelf life because it spoils quickly.

However, if we treat squalene with hydrogen (through a process called "hydrogenation"), we get a saturated form of squalene which is less susceptible to oxygen and, therefore, longer lasting. This hydrogenated state is called "squalane"; it is a more stable, colorless oil with exceptional moisturizing properties. Cosmetic manufacturers use it extensively for making face creams, foundation, eye and hair products, and lipsticks.

The preferred option for cosmetics would be squalane made from olives, as we cannot continue to target sharks for their squalene; slaughtering of sharks for their liver contents is a real concern for environmentalists. According to a study released in 2012 by Bloom, a nonprofit organization, 90% of cosmetics used shark liver oil, contributing to about 2.7 million deep sea shark deaths every year. The Bloom Association said that although Western cosmetic corporations are moving more toward plant-based squalene, the industry is still largely supplied by animal squalene.

The problem today, though, is that not all manufacturers state the origin on the package. Squalane can come from either source; they are chemically identical. But one thing is certain: with such a booming cosmetics industry, the demand for squalane is bound to increase. By checking the label and looking for "vegetable based," "vegetable origins," or "100% plant derived," we as consumers can make sure that we are opting for plant-based squalene instead of animal-based squalene.

A Comparative Study on Olive Oil and Burns

Burns happen when you expose your skin to heat from fire, hot liquids, or to electricity, and occur mostly at home through careless handling of home appliances. You can also be burned by excessive exposure to the sun or through chemicals.

Although you might experience some pain, first-degree burns are relatively minor; they affect mainly the outer layer of the skin, called the dermis. Second-degree burns are a little more serious; they can penetrate to the second skin layer, called the epidermis. With that comes pain and blisters, which need attention. If they're not treated correctly and immediately, second-degree burns can progress to third-degree burns. Third-degree burns are more complicated; that is when the dermis and the epidermis, muscles, tendons, and nerve endings of the area all become damaged.

Researchers conducted studies on patients suffering from second- and third-degree burns using sunflower and olive oil. They wanted to see if consumption of either of these two oils could have an effect on the healing of burn patients. They wanted to know if the healing process could take place internally when taking olive oil orally.

A report published in the journal *Burns* looked at how the body recovered with second-degree burns in a burn care hospital. The study took place on one hundred hospital patients, aged between thirteen and fifty-nine, admitted with burns affecting between 20% and 30% of their body surfaces. They were randomly divided into two groups: one that took extra-virgin olive oil and one that took sunflower oil. They all started taking the oils within twenty-four hours of hospital admission, both groups receiving similar hospital care treatment for their burn conditions—skin grafting, excision of wounds, etc.

Daily examination during their stay allowed the researchers to check and evaluate changes in the surface areas of the burns. They found no significant changes in the body surface of both sets of patients but differences in the duration of wound healing, which ultimately decreased the time spent in the hospital for those taking olive oil.

The authors concluded that "those taking olive oil appeared to have accelerated wound healing and decreased length of stay in the hospital." They added that a larger study involving more patients with more than 20% burn surface taking more olive oil might have more significant results.

Are you wondering how the olive oil made healing faster? The researchers felt that the positive results were due to antioxidants and the anti-inflammatory properties of olive oil.

Olive Oil Solutions

Here are some healthy, safe suggestions for using olive oil at home. We gathered them over time from friends, beauticians, and family. Have fun as you test them.

MORNING DRINK

Wake up the inner beauty in you by starting the day with a lemon, olive oil, and honey concoction. Squeeze the juice of half a lemon into a cup of hot water; add 1 teaspoon of honey and 1 tablespoon of extra-virgin olive oil. Have this before breakfast and make it a routine; it's an ideal way to wake up your liver with a good dose of vitamin C and to start your healthy daily intake of extra-virgin olive oil.

NATURAL EXFOLIANT 1

Our body naturally gets rid of dead skin, but sometimes it hangs on too long, giving us a dull, tired-looking complexion. Exfoliating removes dull, tired, dead cells and rejuvenates the skin. Use this natural scrub twice a week to help keep your complexion clear and healthy. You might need to double the ratios for a whole body and face scrub.

Make a paste using 2 teaspoons of sea salt and 3 tablespoons of olive oil. Using the tips of your fingers, rub the mixture on your face, neck, and body using circular movements, paying special attention to the thicker skin on your knees, elbows, and T-zone area (across the forehead and down the nose forms a T shape). This is also especially good for use on dry, cracked heels.

Natural Exfoliant 2

This sugar exfoliant, a mix of sugar and olive oil, is good for particularly hardened areas, like knees and elbows. Mix equal parts olive oil and sugar into a thick paste, rub it into the hardened areas, leave on for about seven minutes, then wash and dry. Moisturizing after will give you nice smooth skin.

Olive Oil Bath

For all over body smoothness, add a few drops of extra-virgin olive oil to your warm bath.

Makeup Remover

Taking off makeup is less fun than putting it on. If you don't remove all the foundation, mascara, and eyeliner, it clogs up your skin and causes smudges around your eyes. Olive oil, similar in structure to the oils used in makeup, removes all makeup without damaging the skin; it will even get rid of waterproof mascara. Simply dab a little olive oil on a cotton ball and apply over your face and eyes. Rub gently until all the makeup is removed. Rinsing with lukewarm water will remove any residue.

For Shadows and Dark Rings

We sometimes refer to these as bags under the eyes; stress, hereditary factors, and lack of sleep can cause dark circles under your eyes. You'll come across home remedies such as cucumber and tea bags, but did you know you can use a mixture of olive oil and lemon as well?

Mix 2 tablespoons of olive oil with the juice of half a lemon. Using a cotton ball, apply on the eyes, press lightly on the dark circles for about five minutes, then rinse. Lemon is known for its skin-lightening properties, while olive oil hydrates the skin.

MASSAGE OIL

Nothing beats a massage to help you unwind and feel relaxed. Here's massage oil you can use at home. Start by putting 200 millileters (7 ounces) of olive oil in your massage bowl; add the juice of 1 whole lemon and 8 drops or so of lavender oil, the essential oil recognized for its calming and relaxing properties. It is ready to use.

Olive oil is especially beneficial during the winter months when our bodies tend to get really dry. Just remember, though, that it's not the best oil to use on your face as a moisturizer unless you have particularly dry skin.

FACE MASK

We know how important it is to cleanse the face every evening; we do it to remove all the grime and dirt from the day as well as makeup. Every so often, though, we need to go deeper to pull out those impurities that are lurking beneath the top layer of the skin. Using a face mask once a week will do this. It will also unclog our pores and get rid of any pimples caused by bacteria. This healthy, nutritious homemade mask does not take long to prepare; your skin will feel rejuvenated after the treatment. And you get to relax for fifteen minutes while it does its magic.

Mash half an avocado with some olive oil and make into a paste. Smooth it onto your face and leave for about fifteen minutes or so, then rinse.

OLIVE OIL HAIR MASK

Today, the use of too many hair dyes and strong conditioners can cause hair loss. Olive oil has always been used as a natural, effective treatment for hair rejuvenation. Extra-virgin olive oil can be used for the growth, regrowth, and conditioning of hair.

When olive oil or an olive oil product is rubbed into the scalp, the stimulation together with the nutrients from extra-virgin olive oil acts on the hair follicle, penetrating all the way into the hair shaft. As well as providing health supplements, olive oil acts as a barrier to retain the moisture and protect the scalp from the damaging effects of the sun. As a conditioner, olive oil beats any expensive salon treatment.

Heat 3/4 cup of extra-virgin olive oil in a pan or warm in a microwave for a few minutes. Rub into the scalp, continuing right to the ends. Put a towel in the microwave for 2 minutes until it is very warm but not too hot. Wrap around your head for at least 30 minutes to allow the warm oil to penetrate. Wash your hair as normal, using a gentle shampoo.

A Few More Tricks

- To energize a tired face: Mix some olive oil with a few drops of lavender oil and rub onto your face. Cover with a hot flannel and relax for a few minutes.

- To help with wrinkles: Before going to sleep, massage your face with a mixture of oil and lemon juice a couple of times a week.

- To conquer acne: A mixture of olive oil and salt can improve acne if used daily for one week and then two or three times a week after. Mix 5 tablespoons of salt with 4 tablespoons of olive oil, rub the paste onto your face, then rinse off with warm, soapy water.

- To avoid mosquito bites on vacation: Buy some local olive oil, mix with lavender oil and some citronella, and rub on exposed skin.

- To cure an earache and ease irritation of the outer and inner ear: olive oil soothes the ear, opens up the eustachian tubes, and reduces infection. Heat a little olive oil in the microwave for no more than 30 seconds. Apply to the affected ear using an ear dropper and cover with a cotton ball. Repeat if necessary, making sure the oil is not too hot.

- To enhance nail care: Rub a few drops of olive oil into the cuticle area and around the nails for moist cuticles and shiny nails. If you soak your nails once a week in a bowl of lukewarm olive oil for about 10 minutes, they'll become stronger.
- To even a false tan: For a safe, smooth tan, mix equal parts of olive oil with your favorite tanning lotion and apply evenly. Adding olive oil allows the lotion to go on more smoothly and will give you additional moisturizing protection.
- To prevent stretch marks: To avoid stretch marks during pregnancy, apply olive oil two or three times a day and before going to bed.
- To soften scars: Apply olive oil to the scarred areas twice a day; they will disappear in no time.
- To ease diaper rash: Mix 3 teaspoons of olive oil with 1 1/2 teaspoons of water. Wiping baby's bottom with this helps with rashes.
- To prevent fibromyalgia: Fibromyalgia is an arthritis-related condition which causes considerable pain in the muscles and joints. To lessen aches, stiffness, and pain, massage warm olive oil into the affected muscles and joints.
- To ease digestive troubles: Your digestion can be put right with an olive-oil-and-honey combination. Take 1 tablespoon of honey mixed with 1 tablespoon of olive oil in 8 ounces of hot water a couple of times a day.
- For an at-home foot lift: Rub olive oil on your feet before going to bed and then cover with a pair of socks. You'll have nice soft feet in the morning.
- To protect your stomach and liver: If you're going out and planning to have a few drinks, have a tablespoon of olive

oil on a slice of bread before you go. Besides protecting the stomach and liver, olive oil helps delay the passage of alcohol into the bloodstream.

- To substitute for shaving cream: Reach for a bottle of olive oil instead of a bar of soap. Olive oil will glide over your face and legs, moisturizing your skin at the same time.

- To heal slight sunburn: If you've been out too much in the sun, you might feel tenderness with mild sunburn. Mix equal parts of olive oil with water in a lidded container, shake well, and apply on the affected areas of the sunburn.

OLIVE OIL KEEPS BONES HEALTHY

T his is the story of a fifty-seven-year-old, seemingly healthy, retired home economics teacher who suffered a fracture of her spine. It began when osteoporosis caught Susan Smith completely by surprise.

"I fell over while on a walk on frosty grass one day, landed on my back, and expected to suffer somewhat, but I was fine. Four days later, I was out walking again when I tripped on a tree root and fell. The pain started down my back that evening, extreme pain. The doctor didn't seem too worried and put me on painkillers, but I started getting pins and needles in my leg, so I had to go back to the clinic. This time, my doctor ordered X-rays, which showed I had a wedge compression fracture in my spine. Further tests with a DEXA scan confirmed that I had osteoporosis in my spine and osteopenia in my hips. I was in shock! Why did this happen? How did it happen? And why me?"

Susan had to accept that, like many women her age, her bones had become weak and that the osteopenia (low bone density) in her hips was a clear warning that that too could develop into osteoporosis.

The doctor explained why the accident happened.

As her bones aged, it caused the vertebrae of the spine to become weaker; there was too much pressure on the weak spine. As she was five years into menopause, he said, she also had low levels of estrogen, the hormone which regulates the bone cells. These are called osteoclasts and are the cells responsible for building new bones. In short, the vicious cycle of postmenopausal osteoporosis provoking bone loss had started. And it happens to many women as they age— their bone turnover is much faster than men, causing them to suffer more frequently than men from osteoporosis.

Susan lives in the UK, where the incidence of osteoporosis is high. The British Orthopedic Association reports that over 300,000 patients go to hospitals each year with fragility fractures, the type of break you get with osteoporosis. They say most of it relates to hip fractures, resulting in medical and social care costs amounting to £2 billion. The figures are high worldwide. According to data from the World Health Organization (WHO), in 1990, approximately 1.7 million fractures of the femur were recorded in the world and 6.3 million are expected for 2050.

Susan said that after getting over the shock, she started her research, looking closely at what caused osteoporosis, including the importance of getting enough calcium, considered critical for healthy, strong bones. "Now I see that many factors played a part. And some of them I could do nothing about! Above all, I am a woman, I am in my fifties; I can't do anything about my genes, being white, European, with early menopause and a dairy intolerance, and not having had children! Not to mention our modern diet." To her, it seemed like every factor played a part.

But osteoporosis is not just a woman's disease. Statistics show that one in five men over the age of fifty will break a bone mainly due to osteoporosis.

However, statistics also show that people living in the Mediterranean basin following a Mediterranean diet suffered far less from the disease.

As we get old, our bones become weaker, and sadly, there's nothing we can do to stop it from happening. What we can do, though, is slow down the effects of this silent disease by taking in the right nutrients and staying active. Research shows that the antioxidants contained in olive oil have significant positive health benefits on our bones, one way to stay in control and keep osteoporosis at bay.

When we are young, our bone density increases, old bone cells break down, and new cells are constantly being formed. They build strength in our skeletal system. Things change as we get older, however. The turnover does not function as well, more demolition takes place, and we lose our bone strength and become accident prone with greater risks of fractures.

This is the dreaded disease osteoporosis. The disease creeps up on you unexpectedly, often becoming apparent in a dramatic way—usually after a minor injury after a fall. The problem with this disease is that it progresses silently without any signs until we strain ourselves or fall. We develop osteoporosis because, quite simply, our bones have become porous: they no longer have as much strength as they did when we were younger.

A large-scale study in 2013 illustrates this well. The study involving 188,795 people in eight European countries showed that people living in the Mediterranean who stuck to a Mediterranean diet had a lower risk of hip fracture. The bone health of participants—48,414 men and 139,981 women with an average age of forty-six—were followed for over nine years. The researchers in charge of the study assessed the participants' diets and measured how they adhered to the Mediterranean diet. Evaluation at the end of this large study showed only 802 hip fractures for those who adhered to a Mediterranean diet.

According to the study's findings, a Mediterranean eating pattern with high fruit, vegetable, and olive oil intake could be beneficial to improving bone health. But what part does olive oil play?

Scientists in Egypt also wanted to evaluate the protective effects of olive oil supplementation against osteoporosis. To investigate this, they set up comparable situations to female menopause; they wanted to see if olive oil supplements could protect against menopause-induced osteoporosis. In other words, could olive oil prevent bone loss when subjected to similar conditions?

The research was carried out on three groups of rats aged between twelve and fourteen months.

- Group 1: These rats were surgically treated to remove their ovaries.
- Group 2: These rats also received the same surgery. They were given olive oil for a total of twelve weeks: for four weeks before their ovaries were removed and then for eight weeks after the operation.
- Group 3: These rats in the control group did not undergo any operations—they did not have their ovaries removed to induce menopause.

At the end of the experiment, the researchers examined the blood, bones, and livers of all the rats. This is what they found:

- Rats that did not receive olive oil showed a decrease in calcium levels.
- Rats that did not receive olive oil showed an increase in plasma.
- On examination of the blood, the researchers found a lower level of nitrates in Group 2.

More importantly, microscopic examination of the bones of the olive oil–fed rats showed improvement in bone thickness and the ability to replace bone. On comparing the two groups, the researchers said there was a marked improvement in Group 2. They observed that the supplement prevented a decrease in cortical bone thickness as well as the trabecular thickness.

The researchers concluded that olive oil looked like a promising candidate for the treatment of postmenopausal osteoporosis.

Going deeper, we may ask: what components in olive oil were responsible for this sort of result, and can it work on humans?

Researchers at France's National Institute for Agricultural Research (INRA) found the answer. Ranked as the number-one agricultural unit in France, INRA carries out research for high-quality and healthy goods in eighteen centers in France. One of their studies evaluated oleuropein, one of the main components of olive oil.

After their two successful animal trials, the research team at INRA went on to human trials. The aim of this twelve-month study was to measure the effect of taking an olive extract on bone turnover in postmenopausal women with osteopenia, when bone mass had already decreased.

Researchers divided the sixty-four participants who enrolled into two groups. The women, aged between forty-nine and sixty-eight, were all at least twenty-four months past their last menses and all tested, measured, and examined for a number of factors such as weight and cholesterol levels. More relevant, they all had bone mineral density scans at the beginning at the base of the lumbar spine and the neck of the femur using DEXA scans, which were redone and compared at the end of the study.

They were randomly allocated equally between the treatment group and the placebo group. This was a double-blind study where neither the patient nor the investigators were aware of the allocation of the two groups. The test product was an olive extract made up of polyphenols derived from the olive leaf. The researchers were interested in two things: first, they wanted to evaluate the effect of taking an olive oil extract on bone turnover in menopausal women and second, they wanted to study the bone mineral changes and blood lipid profiles.

The study group was given 250 milligrams of olive extract a day (the equivalent of a dose of 100 milligrams of oleuropein per day) as well as 1000 milligrams of calcium. The placebo received 1000 milligrams of calcium with no olive extract.

What they noticed during the study period was an increase in osteocalcin levels in the treatment group. This is what their results showed:

On comparison of the two groups, they found that the levels of osteocalcin increased significantly with the study group as compared with the placebo group. They also found that the bone mineral density decreased in the placebo group but remained stable in the treatment group. Significant, also, was that the lipid levels of the treatment group improved; the total cholesterol, LDL, and triglycerides all decreased.

The researchers concluded from these results that "olive phenolic compounds may have a promising biological activity towards the maintenance of a balanced bone turnover process and blood lipid profile." They said that although this was a limited-scale study, further and larger human-intervention studies could now be set up.

Women and men who suffer from osteoporosis have a fear of something that the rest of us take for granted. They have a fear of crowds—anything from a football match to a crowded theater. Susan, who still battles with osteoporosis, said, "I am afraid to go where there's a crowd. Someone might knock into me and cause my shoulder to break. I am scared of going out in autumn when the leaves are soggy and in winter with ice and snow. Living with osteoporosis can be very hard."

But the results from both studies are encouraging, particularly for women everywhere. There's a factor for osteoporosis prevention and management that we can control just by including olive oil and olive extract in our diet!

OLIVE OIL SLOWS ALZHEIMER'S DISEASE

Our fascinating, complex brain, unlike any other part of the body, has a tight security blood system, a sort of barrier controlling all substances going in and transporting certain molecules out. This blood-brain barrier is like a security fence ensuring proper functioning of the brain by allowing selected molecules and vital elements in; oxygen and essential nutrients can cross over easily. A no-entry mechanism, however, operates for toxins, bacteria, and certain drugs. In a healthy brain, this semipermeable barrier protects the brain, but with Alzheimer's, the circulatory system breaks down, allowing more harmful particles to get inside the brain. And once those harmful particles are in, our healthy brain cells or neurons start producing an abundance of two abnormal structures—two culprits that start disruption.

Imagine losing your memory of your friends and your loved ones and not fully understanding what's going on around you. These are the signs and symptoms of Alzheimer's disease, a disease that clogs the brain, reducing the ability to think, remember, and reason. Drugs can now stabilize the condition, but sadly, once the brain cells are damaged, there's no reversing the damage with this form of dementia. The good news, though, is that researchers have recently discovered that extra-virgin olive oil can help protect the brain from the condition.

Most people associate Alzheimer's disease with old age, but doctors say that even though sufferers may seem normal, damage to the brain can start some twenty years or so before the first symptoms appear. This is a progressive disease, because it takes place gradually over time, contaminating the brain, and as it develops, more symptoms appear, starting mildly and getting worse with time.

The gradual increase in the two abnormal structures accounts for the steady deterioration. The main buildup is caused by clusters of protein fragments called "beta-amyloid" that form outside the neurons. Scientists say these are chemically sticky and so clump up easily to form plaques. The plaques are full of clusters of abnormal tissue that destroy the contact points between the neurons, impeding their communication.

A second unhealthy accumulation also takes place, this time inside the neurons. Twisted fibers of a protein called "tau" develop inside the nerve cells, forming a thick mass known as "neurofibrillary tangles." A healthy brain depends on the correct functioning of the protein tau, but in an unhealthy brain, the tau protein is abnormal and damages the affected brain cells.

These masses of dead and dying cells disrupt the internal transport system of the brain, preventing adequate transportation of nutrients and other essential supplies. With this instability comes a chain of undesirable reactions, from shrinking of the brain to memory loss and lack of communication and reasoning.

Much of the mystery of Alzheimer's has been unraveled since it was first described in 1906. And while the disease affects around thirty million people worldwide, remarkably, people from the Mediterranean countries suffer much less.

Research Studies with Oleocanthal

Research scientist Amal Kaddoumi was raised in Jordan, where the olives are tasty and plentiful, and olive oil is a way of life. She learned of oleocanthal's protective qualities as they were discovered in the scientific world and wanted to delve further to understand why and how the component oleocanthal in olive oil reacted with Alzheimer's disease. Using the brains and cultured brain cells of mice, Dr. Kaddoumi and her team at the College of Pharmacy at the University of Louisiana at Monroe first set out to find out whether the oleocanthal in olive oil was able to reduce the buildup of beta-amyloid, the development of plaques outside the neurons.

Here's how Dr. Kaddoumi explained their findings:

Oleocanthal reduces the accumulation of beta-amyloid in the blood-brain barrier by boosting production of proteins and vital enzymes that are critical for the removal of beta-amyloid. Also, it has an anti-inflammatory effect. However, it's important to use extra-virgin olive oil, as it contains polyphenols, among which is oleocanthal. Refined olive oil lacks these polyphenols and may not show the same effect observed with extra-virgin olive oil.

Encouraged by these results, the researchers then concentrated on a second question: could olive oil then protect us from Alzheimer's?

The second aspect of the study used two approaches: for the first group, the scientists fed mice with extra-virgin olive oil at an age before the amyloid buildup started inside the brain, while the second control group was put on an enriched extra-virgin olive oil diet after the buildup. The results showed that several mechanisms that caused the disease were reduced; most noticeable was a stronger blood-brain barrier and a considerable reduction in the amyloid levels of the first group.

These findings show a definite impact of dietary factors in health, and as Dr. Kaddoumi says, "What we see in animals, we could see in humans." She feels strongly that we can avoid Alzheimer's through healthy eating; a preventive means, she says, would be incorporating extra-virgin olive oil into our daily diet.

Oozing with enthusiasm, she said to us, "These results are exciting. They indicate that oleocanthal and EVOO prevent, or at least delay, the onset of the disease. I recommend people add extra-virgin olive oil, not refined olive oil, to their diet. Oleocanthal is not commercially available, but it is present in extra-virgin olive oil."

Dr. Kaddoumi feels while we wait for more medical evidence, we should include extra-virgin olive oil in our diets as early as possible and that a dose of 50 milliliters (about 3 tablespoons) each day would be a good start. This is the amount they used for their research and what the Greeks would consume daily.

Encouraged by these findings, the team would like to see more studies on humans but realizes the difficulties involved. The team leader explained, "These kinds of studies are costly and require funds. Also, they need to be well designed and controlled to evaluate such effect. We are indeed considering clinical studies, and we are preparing for them. Epidemiological studies also exist; while they don't talk about the mechanism, they showed a positive effect of extra-virgin olive oil on subjects' cognitive function."

Dr. Kaddoumi said she'd like to see more studies and eventual results using a combination of olive oil and other drugs, which she thinks could enhance the effect of the oleocanthal.

Experts will one day hopefully have a deepened understanding of this neurological disorder, which will allow us to nip the disease in the bud. This evidence that extra-virgin olive oil can help combat memory loss and mental decline is positive and encouraging. As life expectancy continues to increase, just think how much money could be saved worldwide every year by families and governments by combating this debilitating disease. The Alzheimer's Association in the United States reports that the illness and other dementias cost the nation $226 billion.

As Dr. Kaddoumi says, "Prevention is the key to protection against Alzheimer's, and the way to do it is to maintain a healthy lifestyle and a healthy, balanced diet. Olive oil is a safe food product accessible to everyone."

Feeding the Brain with the Right Stuff

Numerous studies have investigated the link between the Mediterranean diet and the brain. Briefly, we want to share two studies.

Study 1: We Can Improve Our Memory with Olive Oil and Nuts

A small randomized test conducted in Spain showed that adding a bit more olive oil to a Mediterranean diet might decrease our risk of developing Alzheimer's. Researchers chose older subjects for this study, suggesting that it's never too late to switch to a healthier diet. They selected 447 volunteers between fifty-five and eighty years old, slightly overweight, who had no memory problems but were at a risk of cardiovascular disease. The seniors were assigned to one of three groups: a Mediterranean diet with one liter of extra-virgin olive oil added every week, a Mediterranean diet with 30 grams of mixed nuts added per day, or a low-fat diet. The groups all followed the different diets for four years. All of the members had a total of six cognitive function tests, a series of memory and thinking tests to check their mental state and cognitive changes, before, during, and after the research.

Here are the results as reported by Reuters, the international news agency:

> Based on the brain function tests done before and after the study, the group eating low-fat foods had a significant decrease in memory and cognitive function. The group following a Mediterranean diet with supplemental nuts had significant improvements in memory, while the group adding

extra-virgin olive oil experienced significantly better cognitive function.

This test might be only a small trial, but it does show that monounsaturated fatty acids such as those found in olive oil and nuts present a holistic approach, especially if we want to slow down shrinkage of our brain, prevent the development of plaques, and maintain our cognitive powers. The researchers concluded in their report published in July 2015 that in an older population, a Mediterranean diet supplemented with olive oil or nuts is associated with improved cognitive function.

Study 2: A Look at the Brain Size of Older Seniors

When scientists looked into the eating habits and scanned the brain cells of some older seniors, they found an enormous difference in volume and size between participants.

The aim of the study, as reported in October 2015, was to examine the size of the brain in people who followed a Mediterranean diet "to develop an association." The study involved two groups of people and took place at the same time. The participants who took part had an average age of eighty; some followed a diet aligned more closely with a Mediterranean diet, while others did not.

The 684 older people who came from multiethnic groups in northern Manhattan first answered in-depth questions about their diet and then underwent MRI brain scans to measure the volume and thickness of their brains.

What did the scan results show? Those who followed a more Mediterranean-like diet had a larger brain volume than those who did not. The difference in average brain size was 3.11 milliliters, or the equivalent of five years of aging, the authors reported.

Forgetting where you left the car keys can be considered a mild cognitive behavior, but it could deteriorate into full-blown Alzheimer's with time. As we don't yet know how to target gungy amyloid or the tangles of tau protein—the destructive, deadly duo that comes with Alzheimer's—we can adopt preventive measures to keep them away. The take-home message seems simple: we should incorporate good-quality extra-virgin olive oil to protect ourselves from neurological disorders such as Alzheimer's.

4 Good Reasons for Switching to the Traditional Mediterranean Diet

The Mediterranean diet is the easiest, simplest, most practical diet around, yet in our search for losing weight, we turn to other food plans—the Paleo, the Dukan, and the Atkins diets . . . . The list goes on. However, it is overindulgence of the wrong foods and inactivity that creates the need to lose weight. Wouldn't it be better to incorporate a healthy lifestyle with simple eating—good eating habits that are easy to follow, nutritious, and healthy?

There's no real definition of the Mediterranean diet, no single model. It is more a lifestyle based on a southern European approach that includes food from livestock, fishing, and agriculture. Instead of an excess of meat, the people of the South consume lean sources of protein, drink red wine in moderation, and flavor their dishes with herbs and spices.

The Mediterranean Diet Is Neglected These Days

Sadly, the healthy eating styles and traditions of the Mediterranean diet are being neglected; fast food is gaining popularity, and with that comes the obvious—we are getting fatter. We are all in a hurry these days, not taking the time to choose what we eat, and we're losing the habit of sitting down and enjoying mealtimes.

Those of us who live in the countryside or next to the sea are lucky. It isn't too difficult to follow the Mediterranean diet. The choice of fruit and vegetables is endless in our traditional, open-air markets. Going to the market on Sunday and stocking up on fruit and vegetables is still, thankfully, an essential part of French life.

But here's why we should take a second look at the Mediterranean diet:

MEDITERRANEAN DIET

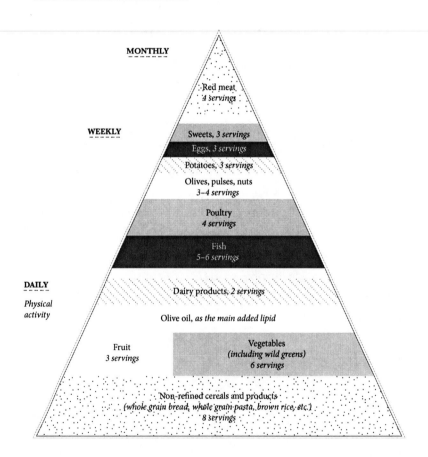

1. NO FOOD RESTRICTIONS

The great thing about the Mediterranean food plan is that there are no strict laws on what we should not eat. Instead, the diet focuses on the variety of fresh vegetables and fruit and encourages us to experiment with locally sourced products. Snacking is not advisable unless, of course, you satisfy those hunger pangs with fresh fruit or nuts. Instead of chips and artificial dips, go for fresh fruit and yogurt.

2. HEALTHY

Originally, this was known as the "Poor Man's Diet" because it did not include much meat—only a bit of fish—and lots of seasonal fruit and vegetables. However, this is the diet that has been proven to reduce heart disease as well as number of medical conditions brought on by the Western lifestyle. This eating plan has been thoroughly researched over the years with scientifically backed evidence showing that you can achieve weight loss and cut back on your risks of certain diseases.

The Mediterranean diet is rich in vitamins, minerals, and fiber and relatively low in saturated fat. It consists mainly of plants, vegetables, fruits, cheese, cereals, and olive oil—the main source of fat. To that, some choose to add one or two glasses of red wine a day (excessive alcohol use can lead to increased risk of health problems), fish, and white meat in moderation and small quantities.

A weekly shopping list would include everything that's healthy, tasty, nonprocessed, and fresh:

- Olive oil is the main fat in Mediterranean cuisine: we cook with it, we have it in salads, and some even use it on bread instead of butter.
- Lots of fruit and vegetables low in fat and high in fiber; popular choices here are zucchini, eggplant, avocados, tomatoes, peppers, and juicy melons.
- Fish packed with protein, vitamins, and minerals.
- Nuts, not to be consumed every day, but two or three times a week.

3. Less expensive

By buying local and fresh, you will not be paying too much for food—especially with a list and a meal plan for the week. Choosing the right food automatically cuts out those costly junk food items. You might be tempted into thinking that it would cost more to go out and buy fresh, but look at what you can cut back on in your current spending; cutting back on those extra soft drinks and cookies is a good way to start. And what about including all the family in the experiment? Planning the meal together could turn out to be a fun activity for the whole family.

4. Balanced lifestyle

The Mediterranean diet is not only about food; it is a lifestyle in which families take the time to eat together—not in front of the television but around the table. It is this sharing which creates a deep appreciation of food.

Considering all the scientific evidence out there as to all of the health benefits the Mediterranean diet has to offer, it makes sense to make the switch. Forget about fad diets; study the Mediterranean diet pyramid, a doable, easy, and versatile plan. Redefining your lifestyle in this way should make you see food as a social interaction with a focus on healthy choices.

It's simple, fresh, wholesome, and, above all, healthy!

OLIVE OIL HELPS REDUCE THE RISK OF DIABETES

A renowned British diabetes specialist noticed that during times of war—when food shortages lead to the removal of white flour, white sugar, and excessive meat protein and fats from the typical British diet—the death rate from diabetes decreased by 50%. If the scientist were still alive, he would be surprised at the healthy eating trend today, the number of food blogs advocating clean, healthy eating, all challenging the way we choose and prepare our meals. And yet diabetes is on the increase. Type 2 diabetes can be managed successfully, however; we need only to choose the right food and exercise more.

We have become much more sedentary these days, spending more time in front of the television. We sit at work. We rely solely on the car to take us places. Many of these factors make us obese, and obesity is one of the reasons we suffer from diabetes. Obesity becomes even more of a problem if we have difficulty controlling our blood sugar levels. Type 2 diabetes has become a worldwide lifestyle disease, which starts when our bodies do not produce enough insulin. It also happens when the cells of our bodies become insensitive to insulin, a condition called "insulin resistance."

Insulin is a hormone produced by the beta cells of the pancreas, the key which unlocks the cells in our bodies to allow glucose in.

Insulin is produced and released when the body needs it; if insulin cannot penetrate into all of the cells in our bodies, then the glucose (blood sugar) gets too high. In type 1 diabetes, the pancreas cannot make insulin, the glucose stays in the blood, and sufferers have to take insulin injections, whereas in type 2, the pancreas produces insulin but it cannot reach the cells.

What's vital to understand is that insulin controls the amount of blood sugar gaining access to our cells; it instructs the body's cells to absorb blood sugar for energy or storage. With type 2 diabetes, our blood glucose levels are high and our insulin sensitivity is decreased. This means that the excess sugar stays in the bloodstream, waiting for insulin activity to kick in so it can get to the cells to provide the energy we so need.

Also important to know is that diabetes has an influence on our good and bad cholesterol. It tends to lower our good cholesterol and raise our bad cholesterol. This combination is not good, because when it happens, we risk having a heart attack or stroke. If left unmanaged, diabetes can also lead to increased susceptibility to cuts and bruises, skin, kidney, and bladder infections, and problems with vision.

But why are we talking about diabetes and cholesterol in a book about olive oil? Because extra-virgin olive oil lowers blood glucose and cholesterol!

A small study was carried out at Sapienza University in Rome, involving only twenty-five participants, all without diabetes. The study looked at the influence diet had on blood sugar in a healthy metabolism. Each of the participants partook of a typical Mediterranean lunch consisting of fish, grains, vegetables, and fruit. They had this meal on two separate occasions; the first time, they added 10 grams (roughly 2 teaspoons) of extra-virgin olive oil to their meal, and the second time, they added 10 grams of corn oil.

They all had their glucose levels measured two hours before and after each meal. The results showed that the glucose levels were much lower after the extra-virgin olive oil meal. The results also showed reduced levels of LDL—the bad cholesterol—with the olive oil meal. On the other hand, the research team found that after the meals with corn oil, the participants had significantly higher LDL levels.

"Lowering blood glucose and cholesterol may be useful to reduce the adverse effects of glucose and cholesterol on the cardiovascular system," said the main researcher. He did stress, however, that he believed it was better to have the olive oil with a meal rather than on its own.

Perhaps, then, if we can lower our level of glucose and LDL, in conjunction with other healthy lifestyle choices, we can prevent the onset of diabetes.

In fact, Spanish scientists from the Institute of Fat in Seville say you can reduce your risk of type 2 diabetes by consuming olive oil. They based their studies on the polyphenol oleic acid in olive oil.

Sergio Lopez, the main researcher, explained that with diabetes, we need to consider the importance of postprandial insulin sensitivity, which he described as a measure of how effectively the body's cells use insulin to reduce elevated blood sugar levels after the ingestion of carbohydrate-containing foods. (The word *post-prandial* means "after a meal.") He said that "appropriate postprandial β-cell function and insulin sensitivity are required to sustain good health." The amount and type of dietary fat are relevant to postprandial response. The researchers said that "oleic acid in olive oil aids to minimize spikes in blood sugar levels after meals by optimizing pancreas production of insulin and improving whole-body sugar utilization."

The researcher also explained that, unlike other dietary fatty acids, such as palmitic acid that you get from some meat and dairy products, oleic acid in olive oil may help to regulate insulin secretion and action in the postprandial state. Monounsaturated fatty acids, then, should be our best choice for the immediate effect of lowering glucose and improving insulin sensitivity in the postprandial state.

According to the World Health Organization (WHO), 90% of people with diabetes around the world have type 2 diabetes. The organization also says that the burden of diabetes can be reduced through prevention by adopting simple lifestyle measures, but not everyone is aware of how lifestyle changes can make a difference. Janet Amos faces that problem in her work as a diabetes specialist nurse.

Amos is based in an inner-city suburb of Manchester in the north of England, an increasingly multicultural population, predominantly from Pakistan and Bangladesh. She says, "My work is more challenging now than ever with an increasing amount of patients with diabetes and prediabetes." At this busy clinic, she sees, on average, between twenty and thirty diabetics each week. Janet says they are very overweight with poor diets and inactive lifestyles.

She explained that patients might come to see her because of a wound that's not healing or an infection that won't go away. They do not understand that the problem is really about shedding their weight, picking the right food, and exercising. What's important and crucial for their health is for her to explain that they are experiencing the effects of type 2 diabetes.

"It is all very challenging," Janet says, "for a health professional trying to get people to change." But it can be rewarding when you see the little changes, like getting them to check their blood regularly and following her advice on food and nutrition. "My greatest reward," she says, "is when I see them controlling their dietary intake and exercising."

Unfortunately, getting her patients to convert to olive oil is often out of the question: the women choose the cheapest oil for cooking, and olive oil is much too expensive for their circumstances.

Growing awareness of the the health benefits of the Mediterranean Diet has led to a rise in olive oil consumption in the United States, but like the UK and rest of the world, diabetes is still a huge problem in the country. We want to share this: the first study conducted outside of the Mediterranean basin and a project to see if higher doses of olive oil would lead to a lower risk of diabetes in the United States.

In the United States, researches from Harvard Medical School and Brigham Young University, working with two Spanish universities, conducted two large cohort studies of 59,930 nurses—aged thirty-seven to sixty-five years from the Nurses' Health Study Group (NHS)—and 85,157 nurses—aged twenty-six to forty-five years from the NHS II group. This was one of the largest studies ever, lasting twenty-two years.

Food questionnaires were sent out every four years. Total olive oil consumption was calculated as a combination of salad dressing olive oil and olive oil added to food or bread. After those twenty-two years, a total of 5,738 cases of diabetes were noted in the NHS group and 3,914 cases in NHS II group.

These are some of the highlights of the study:

- Total olive oil intake was associated with a lower risk of developing type 2 diabetes for participants consuming more than one tablespoon of olive oil per day compared to those who never or almost never consumed olive oil.
- Every additional tablespoon of olive oil was associated with a 6% reduction in type 2 diabetes.
- Replacing one tablespoon of margarine, butter, or mayonnaise with one tablespoon of olive oil was associated with a predicted lower risk of type 2 diabetes. There was a 5% lower risk when replacing margarine with olive oil, an 8% lower risk when replacing butter with olive oil, and a 15% lower risk when replacing mayonnaise with olive oil.

In their report published in August 2015 in the *American Journal of Clinical Nutrition*, the authors concluded that "increased olive oil consumption was associated with a decreased risk of type 2 diabetes."

Olive Leaf and Diabetes

Olive leaf extracts are making the news these days. One of the latest, most interesting studies showed the two main polyphenols in olive oil: oleuropein and hydroxytyrosol. When taken as supplements, these polyphenols can help maintain proper insulin levels. In a twelve-week study that took place in New Zealand, the results showed the effect of these two antioxidants, demonstrating that the duo can improve insulin sensitivity, an exciting promise for those with diabetic risks.

The researchers at Liggins Institute chose forty-six men for the study, aged between forty-one and fifty-one, who were not diabetic but were overweight. Divided into two groups, one group took four capsules of olive leaf extract containing 51.1 milligrams of oleuropein and 9.7 milligrams of hydroxytyrosol daily as a single dose. The other group received the placebo, or a false supplement. Both groups were given capsules, so the identity of what they were taking was completely masked.

After a six-week washout period where both groups did not take any capsules, the researchers switched groups so that those taking the placebo went on the olive leaf supplement while the others also switched to the opposite treatment.

This is what the results showed:

- The olive leaf extract improved the insulin action by 15%.
- The olive leaf extract increased insulin secretion by 28%.

The study concluded that supplementation with olive leaf phenols for twelve weeks significantly improved insulin sensitivity and pancreatic beta cell capacity in middle-aged men, particularly those at risk of developing the group of risk factors, such as elevated blood pressure, which can lead to diabetes.

What's different about olive leaf extract? According to the researchers, olive leaf extract not only increases insulin production but decreases insulin resistance. They reported that olive leaf extract "is a natural product that has an appreciable benefit in improving insulin action in adult overweight males. It worked as well as metformin, the most commonly used diabetes medication in overweight males."

Dr. Martin de Bock, the first author of the paper who conducted the study, answered our question about how oleuropein and hydroxytyrosol—elements in olive leaf extract—can be used as supplements for diabetes:

> There is continuing growth in the nutraceutical industry. It is known that in type 2 diabetes, patients are often more inclined to try alternative medical therapy rather than traditional pharmaceuticals. Therefore, while the incidence of type 2 diabetes continues to increase globally, there is likely to be continued demand for nutraceuticals such as oleuropein and hydroxytyrosol.

Genetics might contribute to type 2 diabetes, but lifestyle, exercise, and diet are things we can change. And we do have that choice today.

Bad Butter

Butter is bad for our health, according to a study funded by the butter industry itself. Amazing but true, this study backfired, showing butter is not as healthy as olive oil.

It is not common that a study commissioned by an industry goes against what they are hoping to promote. Generally, a study such as this one is an excellent marketing tool to improve the image of a product. The results of a study of butter, however, did not give it a good name. The Danish Research Foundation for the dairy operation funded a study on butter in the hope of promoting the image of this lipid.

Instead, it showed that even a moderate intake of butter increases the total cholesterol and LDL in the blood.

The results suggested that hypercholesterolemic individuals—that is, those who have high cholesterol—should keep their butter consumption to a minimum, while the rest of the population could have it as usual, in small quantities, in moderation, raw; in other words, a little butter on toast in the morning is not dangerous.

The study results, published in July 2015 in the *American Journal of Clinical Nutrition*, found that even when consumed in moderation, butter leads to higher cholesterol and LDL in the blood, much more than consumption of alternatives such as olive oil.

What We Should Know about Cholesterol

This waxy substance we sometimes call fat comes from our body. It is made by the liver and circulated through the blood via proteins known as lipoproteins. We also get cholesterol from consuming animal sources like meat and full-fat dairy products. With a diet high in saturated and trans fats, the liver has to produce more cholesterol.

There are two types of cholesterol: the bad cholesterol, LDL (low-density lipoprotein), and the good cholesterol, HDL (high-density lipoprotein). Research shows that when rates are normal and the balance is right, cholesterol protects our arteries by giving them flexibility and strength. Studies also show that HDL recovers the excess cholesterol and carries it back to the liver to be processed before it can be eliminated. LDL carries cholesterol from the liver to all cells. When there is a disruption, LDL cholesterols cause buildup on the walls of the arteries. The buildup accumulates and may contribute to the formation of plaques, which gradually clog the arteries.

Of all cholesterol in the blood, 60–80% is associated with LDL. An increase in bad cholesterol and a decrease in good cholesterol are risk factors which lead to plaque atheroma, causing cardiovascular disease, impotence, and even strokes.

The Composition of Butter

Butter is rich in vitamin A. It also contains vitamin D and vitamin E. With over 730 kilocalories per 100 grams, butter contains 63% saturated fatty acids, 26% monounsaturated fatty acids, and 3.7% polyunsaturated fatty acids. Butter has a low smoke point, which we will talk about in the next chapter, but what's important to know is that this low smoke point of about 177° C (350° F) means that whatever you're cooking will brown and burn quickly, which is bad for your health. All told, butter is probably best taken in moderation—and even better when we only use it raw and for light cooking.

OLIVE OIL HELPS PREVENT STROKES AND HEART ATTACKS

The celebrities in their stunning red dresses parade elegantly down the runway. They were there to present the American Heart Association's "Go Red for Women" Red Dress collection, a colorful event which took place at the department store Macy's in February 2016. The gathering of top models, designers, and celebrities wanted to show their support and to help raise awareness of cardiovascular disease, an illness that affects 44 million women in the United States.

Wearing red for this illness is the obvious choice because red stands out and is the color associated with our hearts. Women suffer more than men from diseases of the heart, and the only way to bring down these high figures is by education. The American Heart Association asks women everywhere to wear red every first Friday in February; it is a ritual they say is beginning to bear fruit, as 90% of women have made at least one healthy behavior change. In the UK, the statistics are also high; the country observes National Heart Month in February as well. With more heart awareness taking place worldwide, women are now checking their cholesterol, increasing their exercise, and making lifestyle changes to prevent cardiac events from happening.

We'd all like our blood to be freely flowing through our bodies, but blood vessels can sometimes get obstructed, and when they do, they can wreak havoc. If blood flow to the brain is not progressing correctly, the body suffers a stroke—a brain attack that disrupts the abilities related to the affected part of the brain; it can come on suddenly, causing numbness, sudden confusion, and dizziness. Strokes occur when a clot (a fatty deposit) blocks the artery in the brain. Equally serious is a heart attack, which causes damage to the heart's muscles when vital oxygenated blood cannot get to those tissues. This, too, is mainly due to a blood clot, blocking the coronary artery supplying blood to the heart. We are familiar with blood clots; we can see the sticky blood cells appear whenever we injure ourselves and form a scab over the cut. That is how the body responds to injury. However, what we do not want are those clots in our blood vessels. The risk factors are the same for strokes and heart attacks: smoking, diabetes, high cholesterol, and high blood pressure, all of which provoke changes in our blood supply system.

In the last chapter, we addressed some of the factors of cholesterol as related to diabetes, but it is perhaps an even more significant risk when considering cardiovascular health. The process that causes the narrowing of the arteries is called "atherosclerosis," said to be caused mostly by the bad cholesterol LDL. All conditions involving the heart and circulation are called "cardiovascular diseases" (CVD), which is one of the leading causes of death in our world today.

You might not be surprised to know that there are fewer incidences of cardiovascular diseases in Mediterranean countries. The American Ancel Keys was the first to study diets, lifestyle, and the incidence of heart disease. On comparing lifestyle and food in seven countries, he found that people living in Greece and Italy who consumed decent amounts of fruit, vegetables, olive oil, grains, and fish were less prone to heart disease than those living in America and Finland, where they ate considerably higher amounts of saturated fats.

You may say the Greeks are noted for adding olive oil to every-thing and that olive oil is fat. You are right; olive oil is a fat, but you know by now that olive oil is a healthy fat. And we must remember, though, that although all types of olive oil are good sources of monounsaturated fats, extra-virgin olive oil offers higher levels of health protection because it is less processed.

Vitamin E, Olive Oil, and Heart Disease

Interesting in the fight against cardiovascular disease were the results of a study carried out on women in Naples, Italy. It showed that women who consumed more vitamin E were less likely to show signs of heart disease. The women taking part in the study did not take any additional supplements of vitamin E nor did they have any special dietary recommendations for the study. They simply followed their normal Mediterranean way of life; in other words, they continued having their usual regimen of legumes and vegetables, together with olive oil. On examination with ultrasound, these women showed little trace of thickening in the carotid arteries of the neck, an accepted medical marker for vitamin E in the body.

Three hundred and ten women, aged between thirty and sixty-nine years old, took part in the study. All the women had ultrasound tests to see whether they showed early signs of atherosclerosis in their carotid arteries. They had additional blood tests as part of the study to check their levels of vitamin E, other antioxidants, and cholesterol.

In their results, published in the *American Journal of Clinical Nutrition*, the researchers said that the "more vitamin E the women consumed, the less likely they were to show signs of atherosclerosis." They also found that additional vitamin E only helps those who start off with low amounts and that those with sufficient amounts of vitamin E would not benefit from increasing their amount. It also seems that the other antioxidants present in olive oil—vitamins A and C—did not have an effect on carotid thickening.

Why You Should Look at Vitamin E More Closely

We've mentioned vitamin E briefly in several sections because this little-known vitamin is so beneficial to the body. Why is it so important?

Vitamin E was first discovered in Berkeley, California, by two scientists who were exploring infertility in female rats. The scientists could not understand why the pups were dying in their mothers' wombs; something was obviously missing from the diet they were being fed. The scientists eventually discovered that a diet of lettuce and wheat germ resolved the problem; it seemed that a compound contained in both substances was the answer. With time, they were able to isolate vitamin E successfully.

Here are some of the most significant things to know about vitamin E:

- Vitamin E contains eight different compounds that make up the vitamin E family; each of these is fat soluble and can be found in food substances. They are all similar except for a simple difference of molecular structure.
- Olive oil contains alpha-tocopherol, the most common and the most efficient of the eight compounds.
- Vitamin E is the best antioxidant for fighting free radicals. Our brain cells, in particular, are more susceptible to damage from free radicals; it is vital that they are protected.
- The heart needs vitamin E. The vitamin acts on LDL, the bad cholesterol, limiting oxidation. LDL oxidation accelerates the building up of plaques within our arteries (see page 100).
- Although the heart and the brain do need more protection, all of the cells of our bodies also need constant protection; the cell membranes and the tissues of the skin,

eyes, breast, liver, and testes all benefit from the antioxidant properties of vitamin E.

- Besides olive oil, you can get vitamin E from nuts, green vegetables, and vegetable oils.
- According to the IOC, it is important to maintain correct levels of vitamin E during breastfeeding. Women need more vitamin E during pregnancy, as the vitamin is concentrated in the breast. When they breastfeed, mothers supply essential nutrients, vitamin E in particular, to the newborn baby.

Oxidative Stress and Antioxidants

If you leave a coin out in the open for some time, the rain, the sun, and other environmental factors will cause it to go green and rust, a process called oxidation. This interaction between oxygen molecules and outside substances is a normal process. A very similar process takes place in the cells of our bodies; the oxidative process can also cause destruction and havoc to our bodies.

Much of the damage is caused by free radicals. Often labeled as harmful products, they invade our immune system. They are called free radicals because these molecules roaming around our bodies are unstable; unlike other normal molecules, which exist in pairs, they lack one electron. In their search to become stable, they seek to react with other molecules looking for stability. Free radicals will continue to circulate in the system as long as the body continues to function and age. Scientists say not all free radicals are harmful, but when there are lots of free radicals in the body, it becomes dangerous for our health. Our bodies can only take on so many roaming radicals. When there is too much buildup, the body suffers.

What causes this buildup? Some of the most common causes are smoking, pollution, drugs, too much exposure to sunlight, radiation, and stress. The body suffers from oxidative stress when too many free radicals are produced, causing damage to the cells of our bodies by the oxidative process. Scientists say oxidative stress can cause a plethora of undesired human pathologies, such as Parkinson's disease, diabetes, rheumatoid arthritis, cancers, and heart diseases.

Thank goodness for antioxidants, man-made or natural substances that donate electrons that these free radicals need, such as vitamin E. Antioxidants fight and neutralize the reaction, allowing the body to function normally—in other words, by intervening, they stop the oxidation process by oxidizing themselves.

Although the body produces some antioxidants, with the increase in pollution and lifestyle demands, we need other, outside sources of antioxidants, healthy foods that will provide a healthy balance of oxidants and antioxidants. Olive oil contains some key polyphenols recognized as natural antioxidants, particularly vitamin E.

Research into Olive Oil and Heart Conditions

Today, there are numerous case-controlled studies of the Mediterranean diet showing the protective benefits of olive oil. Researchers are also continuously investigating the influence of olive oil on cardiovascular diseases; dedicated scientists from different parts of the world all use various methods, but with one aim—discovering how to improve our heart health.

Although anyone of any age can suffer a heart or brain attack, most sufferers are over sixty-five years of age. One of the first studies to look at the effect of olive oil and the risk of stroke took place in France. It lasted six years and involved 7,625 participants aged over sixty-five. Led by Cécilia Samieri from the University of Bordeaux and the National Institute of Health and Medical Research (INSERM), the primary aim of the large-scale study was to investigate the relationship between olive oil consumption and the risk of stroke in older subjects. The seniors taking part came from different regions in France: Montpellier in the south, Bordeaux in the southwest, and Dijon in central France.

They were all interviewed at the start of the study to make sure they did not have any existing heart condition and also to determine how much olive oil they consumed in general. The researchers then formed three groups based on the three levels of olive oil consumers:

- Group 1 (23%): those who never used olive oil
- Group 2 (40%): those who used it moderately for cooking, salad dressings, and with bread
- Group 3 (37%): those who used it intensively for cooking, salad dressings, and with bread

More interviews and questionnaires followed two, four, and finally six years after the baseline visit.

The final results showed the following:

- A total of 148 suffered strokes.
- Participants in Group 3, who used olive oil regularly for cooking and salad dressings, had a 41% lower risk of stroke compared with those who used none.
- The overall stroke rate was 1.5% for olive oil users compared to 2.6% for the participants in Group 1.

At the conclusion of the study, Samieri said that since stroke was so common in older people, olive oil would be an inexpensive and easy way to help prevent it.

This was a well-designed cohort study (a study over time); however, it was an observational study, not a randomized study where some of the subjects took olive oil and others didn't. It was based on responses from the participants making their own assessments. And, as it took place throughout different regions of France, the other food could have varied considerably. Another factor which could have influenced the result is that for whatever reason, people sometimes change their eating habits. We do not know what type of olive oil the participants used—be it expensive extra virgin or a cheaper option—but their eating habits relating to olive oil could have changed during the study.

Study in Spain

A second and more rigorously controlled study which took place in Spain showed more conclusive and clear results. In the PREDIMED study (Prevention con Dieta Mediterránea), participants changed their diet and were subjected to stricter methods of control than the French study.

The main aim of the Spanish study was to show the effects of the Mediterranean diet as a primary prevention of cardiovascular disease. It involved people with high risk factors but who had not yet developed the disease. The study wanted conclusive evidence as to whether or not the Mediterranean diet supplemented with nuts or extra-virgin olive oil could prevent strokes or cardiovascular disease–related deaths in comparison with a low-fat diet.

This was also a large-scale study; a total of 7,447 participants took part in the five-year study. Although none of the men (aged between fifty-five and eighty years old) and women (aged between sixty and eighty years old) had a history of cardiovascular disease at the time of enrollment, they were all at high risk of heart attacks and strokes. To be selected for the study, they had to have either type 2 diabetes or at least three risk factors such as smoking, hypertension, low good cholesterol (HDL), high bad cholesterol (LDL), being overweight, or having a strong family history of heart disease.

- Group 1 stuck to their normal Mediterranean diet, which encourages red wine but limits red meat, soft drinks, and commercially baked products. They received extra-virgin olive oil weekly and were instructed to have as much olive oil as they could—at least 1/4 cup per day.
- Group 2 continued their normal Mediterranean diet but with an increase of nut intake. They, too, were given weekly

supplies and were told to eat at least 1/4 cup of unsalted mixed nuts daily: 15 grams of walnuts, 7.5 grams of hazelnuts, and 7.5 grams of almonds.

➨ Group 3 participants were advised to follow a low-fat diet and were told to limit their intake of olive oil and nuts.

After nearly five years, of the 7,447 participants, 288 suffered one of three endpoint events—heart attack, stroke, or death from a cardiovascular cause. The results showed that those assigned to the Mediterranean diet plus olive oil had a 30% reduced risk of a combined endpoint of heart attack, stroke, and cardiovascular death. (Interestingly, the study also showed that those who followed the Mediterranean diet displayed a noticeable reduction in belly fat.)

One of the major limitations of the study was that it focused only on Spanish people, who have a common culture. Professor Salas Salvado explained: "It's hard to extrapolate our results to other populations. This is a limitation of inherence to all clinical trials. First, we need to clarify in the future if adherence to the Mediterranean diet is achievable in other non-Mediterranean countries."

He explained that some ingredients (particularly olive oil) are difficult to find in some countries, or some (like wine) are forbidden for religious reasons. He said that some cultural differences in cooking might make it difficult to adopt a traditional Mediterranean food pattern.

However, despite the limitations of the study, Professor Salvado said: "For the first time, a scientific study of large scale could demonstrate the efficiency of the Mediterranean diet in primary prevention cardiovascular pathologies."

The researchers concluded: "In summary, we found that greater consumption of total olive oil, especially extra-virgin olive oil, was associated with reduced cardiovascular disease and mortality risk in an elderly Mediterranean population at high cardiovascular risk. Our findings underscore olive oil consumption as one of the key components of the Mediterranean diet for cardiovascular disease prevention."

The PREDIMED researchers said that 50 grams (about 3.5 tablespoons) of extra-virgin olive oil is the best dose for a person at high risk of cardiovascular disease and that the incidence of the disease can be reduced by 10% for every 2 teaspoons.

Study in Scotland

The two studies above demonstrate the link between diet and health in older subjects, but both long-term studies took a long time to gather enough data for analysis. However, a study conducted in 2014 in Glasgow, Scotland, showed a new way to measure subtle changes in the heart. The good thing about their method is that it takes only a few weeks to see results. The research study involves proteomics, a science which looks at protein patterns in the urine.

Unlike the PREDIMED study involving three different groups, including the control one, all of the volunteers in Glasgow took olive oil (some with high phenolics, while others took low-phenolic olive oil). Researcher Dr. William Mullen of the Institute of Cardiovascular and Medical Sciences said this was the first time proteomics was used from a nutritional perspective and that one of the aims of the research was to show which food was truly responsible for health benefits. The conclusions of the study would influence more accurate labeling, he said, and allow informed consumer choice. Dr. Mullen stated that the main target for their studies was to provide a means to test whether certain health foods—in this case, olive oil—do in fact have a beneficial effect on heart disease. At present, he said there were no standardized tests to assess foods for heart health benefits.

How does the test work? Our urine contains not only waste products but also medical evidence that can tell us what is happening inside our bodies. These are proteins which allow scientists or doctors to work out a "protein fingerprint" for different diseases. The study uses urinary biomarkers (measured biological evaluation) as a sort of reporter for the detection of illnesses before the damage starts appearing. Dr. Mullen said that other sorts of research are limited; for example, we can measure cholesterol to get an idea of your risk of heart disease, but it does not tell you if you have the disease. In other words, we might be pleased to see our printed laboratory results indicating normal cholesterol levels, but it cannot show an existing heart disease that's totally unrelated to our cholesterol levels.

For the study, researchers chose sixty-three healthy volunteers from Glasgow, participants who did not take olive oil regularly (the Scottish are not big consumers of olive oil). Aged between eighteen and seventy-five years old, the participants were medically screened before being accepted. None of them suffered from chronic diseases of the gastrointestinal tract, were on any form of medication, or had taken any recent antibiotics. The group included smokers as well as nonsmokers but excluded pregnant and lactating women.

This was a double-blind study where neither the subjects nor the research team knew which oil the participants were taking. Participants were randomly divided into two groups: one group that took extra-virgin olive oil with high phenols and another group that took normal olive oil with lower phenols. During the study time, they all had 20 milliliters of olive oil from Portugal as a daily supplement, but the oils were not heated or used in cooking. There were no dietary restrictions; they simply took the oil at any time during the day at a single intake.

The researchers used a scoring system, with all the healthy participants beginning with an equal score. Urine samples were taken at the beginning of the study, analyzed, and given a "below-the-disease threshold" baseline score of 0.14. At the end of the first three weeks, each urine sample was again analyzed and given a score for its protein characteristic followed by a calculation of the average heart disease score. This was repeated at the end of six weeks.

The results revealed that the average measure of coronary artery disease for both groups decreased. The researchers said that after three weeks, those on low-phenolic oil showed a decline in the score of 0.3 while the group on the high-phenolic oil showed a score of 0.2. Interestingly, urine analyses at the end of the study did not reveal any significant differences between the two groups; in other words, any olive oil, low or high in phenolics, seemed to be beneficial.

The researchers concluded that although there was an improvement in scores for coronary artery disease, there was no significant contribution of olive oil phenolics. They said that in the population studied, "any olive oil high or low in phenolics seems to be beneficial, and . . . the fatty acids were probably the main contributors to the observed effect."

The beauty of this test is that it can be used to quickly confirm what foods are good for health so that the public can make informed choices about the food they include in their diet. Dr. Mullen said that identifying the early signatures of disease before they become a problem would considerably reduce medical intervention. The results, he added, could have a real, positive impact on the health of the general public, and if people in the UK reduced part of their fat intake with olive oil, it could have an even greater effect on reducing the risk of heart disease.

When asked about what the results might mean in the future, the researcher was optimistic: "We were very excited about the results of this study, as it provided evidence that, using a relatively small sample size of volunteers over a relatively short intervention period, we could provide statistically significant proof of a benefit in heart health in the general population."

If proteomics could be used to measure the health effects of certain foods, the conclusions would indeed be an incentive for people to change their diet because they would be able to see the results. In the long run, that would reduce the high healthcare costs, estimated at up to £11 billion in the UK. The economic burden of CVD, including indirect costs from premature death and disability, is estimated to be over £15 billion each year in the country.

Can Canola Replace Olive Oil for a Healthy Heart?

Making the cooking news these days is the vegetable oil canola, also called "rapeseed oil." Suddenly, canola oil is big business, and some say that it can replace olive oil. These two oils are, however, quite different. Olive oil comes from a long history. It is steeped in tradition, while canola oil is relatively new.

Rapeseed oil is made by crushing the seeds of the rapeseed plant. For this, they use high temperatures, and during manufacture, solvents and chemicals are added. Olive oil, on the other hand, comes straight from the olive fruit; it is pure juice, usually cold pressed without using heat and solvents during extraction.

What's important to consider for health reasons is their stability when we use them for cooking; in other words, how resistant are they to oxygen? This is vital, as you do not want too many chemical changes taking place while cooking; you want to avoid oxidation, a reaction with the air. Consider the smoke point of the oil, the temperature at which the cooking oil or fat breaks down. When heated, olive oil is one of the most stable, principally because it is rich in monounsaturated fats. The smoke point of canola varies according to the variety and growing conditions.

The International Olive Council says the following:

Olive oil in proper temperature conditions, without overheating, undergoes no substantial structural change and keeps its nutritional value better than other oils.

When heated, olive oil is the most stable fat, which means it stands up well to high frying temperatures. Its high smoke point (410° F or 210° C) is well above the ideal temperature for frying food (356° F or 180° C). The digestibility of olive oil is not affected when it is heated, even when it is reused several times for frying.

(This statement refers to extra-virgin olive oil; the cheaper brands have lower smoke points.)

The *British Journal of Nutrition*, after studying the health benefits of both oils, said the evidence for the protection afforded by extra-virgin olive oil is "convincing" but that evidence for canola oil was short term and that it is prone to oxidation when frying.

Extra-Virgin Olive Oil Reduces Blood Clots

We've addressed that clots block the arteries carrying blood and that people in the Mediterranean seem to have fewer attacks. But is this because olive oil affects the blood's ability to form clots? If we could control clotting in the blood, then perhaps we could reduce the vast number of heart attacks.

In Denmark, at the Royal Veterinary and Agricultural University, Frederiksberg scientists looked at how blood clots react with different oils. Researchers wanted to compare the effects of extra-virgin olive oil, rapeseed oil, and sunflower oil on the blood coagulation factor VII. They recruited healthy subjects for this study: eighteen fit young men who ate diets with high contents of olive oil, rapeseed oil, or sunflower oil. After three weeks, when they checked the levels of factor VII of each group, they found that the readings were considerably lower for those on the diet rich in olive oil as compared to those on the sunflower and rapeseed oils.

It does not take a long time for a clot to form in an artery and stop the flow of nourishment from getting to the brain and heart. Risk factors like age and heredity we cannot control, but we can choose to replace saturated fats with monounsaturated fat in our diet. Choosing a healthy diet such as the Mediterranean diet coupled with regular exercise helps keep the interior walls of our blood vessels free to pump blood to our hearts, the way it should be.

PART III

Understanding the Label and Buying Extra-Virgin

Once you understand the label, buying extra-virgin olive oil becomes easy.

How often have you stood in front of a row of extra-virgin olive oils, bewildered by the choices and confused by the labels? Don't worry; you are not alone. The wording that manufacturers use is not always easy to follow, and the bottles come in various sizes and different colors, some with impressive-sounding labels. Mandatory information such as provenance, quantity, and company brands are clear, but how can we be sure of the quality of the contents? What does "light olive oil" mean?

As consumers, we scrutinize the label because we want to buy the best olive oil, especially now that we are more aware of the health benefits and the organoleptic aspects of extra-virgin olive oil. Buying the right olive oil, however, is not easy these days because of complicated phrases and confusing terminology, and besides, we are put off by the alarming increase of fraud in the olive oil world.

Phrases like "packed in Italy" or "bottled in Italy" do not mean that the oil was made in Italy or that it was made from Italian olives. Often, too, a label claiming that the oil is extra virgin is nothing but cheaper oil sold at the same price as good-quality extra-virgin olive oil or, even worse, cheaper, low-grade oil blended with refined olive oil and passed off as fresh olive juice.

To safeguard against these fraudulent practices and to protect the consumer, The International Olive Council has enforced strict standards for their member countries, which account for 98% of the world's olive oil supply. Most non-IOC members also have established norms and practices to ensure that the contents live up to what the label says, particularly regarding chemical and organoleptic standards.

Things were different a few years ago when olive oil was mostly a Mediterranean product and a Mediterranean way of life, but extra-virgin olive oil has become a global product present in 150 countries. Because of the considerable increase in olive oil consumption with new markets and new producers all over the world, it is important to protect consumers with common regulatory statements: compulsory declarations relating to bottling and selling all types of olive oil everywhere.

If you can, it's best to buy from a reputable producer, but this is not always possible. That is why it is vital to study the label, paying close attention to the compulsory statements; it is the best guarantee that you are getting the real thing.

Look for Two Magic Words: "Extra Virgin"

Ignore any bottles labeled "100% pure olive oil," "light olive oil," or any similar terminology. Pick up, instead, one which says "extra virgin." These two words tell you that this is the highest grade of olive oil, that it was made without any added chemicals, and that that the producer took extra care during the extraction process to keep the temperature at 27° C or lower. This is sometimes labeled as "first cold pressure." It means that you are getting the maximum nutritional and organoleptic qualities. Heat matters because although excessive heat yields more oil, the quality becomes inferior when processed this way. "Extra virgin" on the label also tells us that only the best olives were used, that the oil was laboratory tested, and that it meets the required chemical and organoleptic standards. It is in the best commercial category approved by the IOC.

Following closely behind the extra virgin category is the description, also a mandatory statement from the IOC:

> Virgin olive oils are the oils obtained from the fruit of the olive tree solely by mechanical or other physical means under conditions, particularly thermal conditions, that do not lead to alterations in the oil, and which have not undergone any treatment other than washing, decantation, centrifugation, and filtration.

Check the Dates

The second important thing you should look for is the "best before" date or the "harvesting" date. Shelf life can be variable, and though some producers might give an optimal "use by" date or say "preferentially to two years," a lot depends on the olive variety. The harvesting date is probably most useful for consumers, but bear in mind that you need to think about how the oil was stored in the supermarket, a factor which plays an important part in the lifespan of olive oil. Remember that the younger the oil, the better it is for your health. Don't buy oil that is more than eighteen months past harvest time. Getting one from this year's harvest is the best proof of freshness.

Check the Origin of the Olives

The label is a kind of contract between the producer or the bottling enterprises and the consumer. The source of the fruit and the geographic region for some consumers serve as a guarantee of quality; these days, consumers like to see the clear, direct path right up to the production process. However, if the identification of the supplier is necessary, the origin of the fruit is not always mentioned. In most cases, the supplier is not the person who owns the olive plantation. Take, for example, the case of Italy, one of the world's major importers of olive oil. You might be surprised to learn that much of the fruit comes from orchards in Spain, Greece, and Tunisia. Also, Italians consume some of the oil imported into Italy, but much of it is blended, packed, and re-exported. Legislation laws in Europe now protect consumers with a more detailed traceability chain, with regulations that stipulate that either the origin of the olives or the place of harvesting be mentioned on the label.

Look for the Certification

Although rules and regulations concerning certification vary from country to country, here's what you need to know.

Are you buying olive oil from Europe?

The United States is the second biggest importer of olive oil (after the EU), and, not surprisingly, most of the olive oil sold in the United States comes from Europe. Certification on the label is the best guarantee that your olive oil comes from where it says on the bottle.

A Protected Designation of Origin (PDO) on the label is the European certificate that confirms that the product comes from a particular European country. This means that the olive oil was produced and processed in the same place. If your oil comes from Europe, it may carry one or two of the following:

- AOC: The French term for PDO is *Appellation d'Origine Controlée.*
- DPO: The Italian version of PDO is *Denominazione d'Origine Protetta.*
- PGI: Protected Geographic Indication. This shows that at least one stage of production, processing, or preparation took place in the geographic location.

The benefits of olive oil can now be highlighted through labeling and marketing. The European Food Safety Authority (EFSA) allows the following health claim on extra-virgin olive oil labels: "Olive oil polyphenols contribute to the protection of blood lipids from oxidation stress." The European Commission stipulates, however, that the claim may be used only for olive oil which contains at least 5 milligrams of hydroxytyrosol and its derivatives.

Are you buying olive oil from the United States?

Although federal standards are very similar to the IOC, these are only voluntary and not mandatory.

If you are buying from the United States, look out for the following:

- The COOC Seal: This is the California Olive Oil Council seal, which shows that the oil has passed both the chemical and sensory tests to be sold as extra-virgin olive oil.
- The NAOOA Seal: The North American Olive Oil Association seal shows that the oil was imported and meets IOC standards. Many leading brands in the retail industry carry this seal.

Interestingly, you may see the following claim on an olive oil bottle, allowed since 2004 by the United States Food and Drug Administration (FDA):

Limited and not conclusive scientific evidence suggests that eating 2–3 tablespoons (23–50 grams) of olive oil daily may reduce the risk of coronary heart disease due to the monounsaturated fat in olive oil. To achieve this possible benefit, olive oil is to replace a similar amount of saturated fat and not increase the total number of calories you eat in a day. One serving of this product contains [x] grams of olive oil.

Storing Extra Virgin

You've carefully selected your precious green nectar, but how do you store it?

Don't save it for special occasions! Contrary to wine, olive oil does not get better with time. Extra-virgin olive oil is freshly squeezed fruit juice—it's seasonal, perishable, and best at its freshest (within the first week of pressing). As with all fresh food products, both the taste and the aroma of olive oil lose quality with time. The overall quality starts deteriorating just a few months after milling, declining rapidly when the oil is bottled and even faster when the bottle is opened.

That is why it is increasingly common to have recommendations or advice on how to store your olive oil on the label.

Here's what you should know:

Auto-oxidation and photo-oxidation are the two culprits responsible for causing the oil to oxidize. Unlike other cooking oils, extra-virgin olive oil contains natural antioxidants, which protect it somewhat from auto-oxidation (oxidation that occurs in the presence of oxygen). It is, however, very sensitive to photo-oxidation (oxidation caused by light). To avoid your extra virgin going bad, store the oil away from light, heat, and air (oxygen). A sealed bottle of extra-virgin olive oil lasts between nine and twenty months, but once opened, it is best to use it up within three months. Although the oil is still okay to use, oxidation might cause an unpleasant odor and taste. More importantly, the sensory and nutritional qualities start diminishing rapidly.

To limit oxidation and to conserve your extra virgin, you should ideally keep your bottle between 15° C and 20° C (59–68° F). The following is advisable:

- Store the bottle in a cupboard away from direct light, such as from a window. You need to protect it from ultraviolet rays.

- It might look pretty in a clear bottle, but choose a tinted glass container. Also suitable is a nonreactive metal such as stainless steel.
- You should not use plastic. Although it is light, plastic is porous and lets in light, air, and humidity as well as ultraviolet rays.
- Heat is just as dangerous when it comes to storing olive oil. Keep it away from any heat source such as above the oven or stove.
- Try to buy your oil in small amounts, ideally in containers of about 250 or 500 milliliters (1 or 2 cups), or transfer it to smaller containers to use for the week.

Remember: olive oil starts degrading quickly, so cover it immediately after each use. You could invest in an olive oil pourer; they come with long metal spouts, ideal for continuous pouring. If you can get a ceramic or stainless steel one, that's even better; it will keep the light out, thus protecting your oil from oxidation.

DIFFERENT CATEGORIES OF OLIVE OIL

With growing awareness, new research, and concerns for our health, the Mediterranean basin is no longer the only center of olive oil production. The demand for the olive fruit is growing, with about eighty-six liters of olive oil produced every second in the world. Unfortunately, not every liter produced is real, natural juice; only two categories can be classed and sold as pure olive oil.

To ensure quality standards in olive oil production, the International Olive Council has established very specific regulations for all types of olive oil. To make it easier for the consumer, we focus here on the most common categories, those we find in supermarkets. To understand the complexity of this product, we have added at the end of this chapter the ten categories of olive oil defined by the IOC as well as those of the United States. These are somewhat similar but aren't compulsory for producers in the United States.

Before bottling, the producer or the person in charge of the commercialization must submit a sample of his oil for testing. Based on the results of physicochemical tests and sensory test, the oil will be assigned a category. This is where the story gets complicated, because the classification of olive oils is anything but simple.

The first family of olive oils extracted exclusively from olives by mechanical or physical processes is called "virgin olive oil." Any other oils obtained using solvents, high temperatures, or any mixture with oils of other kinds are excluded from this category.

Extra-virgin olive oil is obviously the most superior olive oil, the best quality you can get. As production methods are carefully surveyed, the oil retains all its nutritional and aromatic properties. It is a pure fruit juice, just as fresh and nutritious as freshly squeezed orange juice. The label often includes the phrases "first cold pressed" or "extracted cold," which signifies that this was the first time the fruit was extracted and that the temperatures during the mixing stage did not exceed 27° C (80.6° F).

According to the criteria of the IOC, extra-virgin olive oil must meet three quality settings: it must have a low acidity (below 0.8%), a nice, pleasant aroma that reminds us of healthy fruit (such as the olive or another similar fruit or vegetable), and no sensory defects such as fermentation or oil rancidity.

If the chemical test for acidity of the oil exceeds 0.8%, it will be noted as having a slight defect; the oil then gets put in the "virgin olive oil" category, still classed as first cold-pressed oil but with a slight defect which the consumer does not always notice. The acidity is a chemical parameter that shows the freshness and quality of the oil; it is not something that the consumer or the professional taster can distinguish. A low acidity shows that manufacturing was carried out in optimum conditions and in a very short time between harvest and pressure, with natural and mechanical methods, without chemical additives.

Why does acidity exceed the limit?

The virgin olive oil, from the tree to bottling, may suffer some alterations of fruit or oil. The 2014–2015 harvest in some parts of Europe, for example, was catastrophic due to unfavorable climate conditions: a rainy summer and a mild winter that caused an invasion of olive flies. These flies lay their eggs directly on the fruit, allowing the larvae to feed on the flesh of the olive. From the outside, it is difficult for a grower to see the larvae; only the extracted oil with a high acidity reading, as well as an unpleasant taste in the mouth and nose, will tell. The oil cannot be consumed in this state and must be refined before it can be sold.

Some other factors can damage the fruit and oil. The list is long but includes very long storage of the fruit before extraction, using fruit that fell to the ground, diseases, prolonged contact with oil and organic materials, and temperatures being too high during malaxing.

According to IOC regulations, if a virgin olive oil has acidity above 2% or a marked sensory defect, it becomes lampante oil and cannot be sold for consumption. Growers strive for low acidity levels; they do not want to see their oils downgraded and sent to the refinery.

Let's now consider the second family. These are virgin olive oils with defects or second-pressed oils. Pressing a second time extracts another 3%–8% of oil that could not be obtained from the first press.

These oils cannot be sold and are sent to the refinery to be chemically treated. This process removes all the smell, taste, and color. Although the first press renders a natural product, the second is an industrial product that has nothing to do with fruit juice.

This classification makes it tough for the consumer. Education and promotion are essential for extra-virgin olive oil. It is the only natural juice—the only one which has all the health benefits and endless cooking options.

The second challenge for the International Olive Council is the harmonization of quality standards for consumer countries which are not producers, such as Brazil and China. Issues today concern protection from fraudulent practices (such as the mixing of olive oil with other vegetable oils or the sale of a lower quality at the price of extra-virgin olive oil, for example). Strangely, it's an increasingly regulated sector and often quoted in the press for fraud.

A few years ago, olive oil was mostly a Mediterranean product and a Mediterranean way of life; this is no longer the case. Extra-virgin olive oil has become a global product, present in 150 countries all over the world. Consumption is increasing in nonproducer countries, too. According to the IOC, the United States is the biggest importer of olive oil, followed by these nine countries: Brazil, Italy, Japan, China, Canada, Australia, Russia, Spain, and Switzerland. Nonmember countries account for 82% of the worldwide imports.

Food products must have a label that complies with the legislation of the country where they will be sold and distributed. The information supplied guarantees health protection and also protects consumers against fraud. These rules of labeling and classification of oils, according to chemical and organoleptic parameters, must be applied by all member countries of the International Olive Council, which carry 98% of world production. How else can we be sure that the contents are the same as what it says on the label?

Rules to protect the consumer in nonmember countries vary from country to country.

Mandatory Standards

For nonmember countries, the legislation to protect the consumer varies according to the country and each competent institution. The International Olive Council is working closely with the Codex Alimentarius to homogenize the mandatory standards.

Some nonmember countries, like Brazil and Japan, work closely with IOC. With such collaboration, these countries are gradually adopting the official standard. In the United States, the federal standard is voluntary, not mandatory, but very similar to the IOC's guidelines. In Australia, the Australian Olive Association, which represents Australian growers, sets and maintains quality standards through the Code of Practice (COP).

Designations and Definitions of Olive Oils from the International Olive Oil Council

Virgin olive oils are the oils obtained from the fruit of the olive tree (*Olea europaea L.*) solely by mechanical or other physical means under conditions, particularly thermal conditions, that do not lead to alterations in the oil, and which have not undergone any treatment other than washing, decantation, centrifugation, and filtration. Virgin olive oils are fit for consumption.

- Extra-virgin olive oil: virgin olive oil which has a free acidity, expressed as oleic acid, of not more than 0.8 grams per 100 grams, and the other characteristics of which correspond to those fixed for this category in the IOC standard.

- Virgin olive oil: virgin olive oil which has a free acidity, expressed as oleic acid, of not more than 2 grams per 100 grams and the other characteristics of which correspond to those fixed for this category in the IOC standard.

- Ordinary virgin olive oil: virgin olive oil which has a free acidity, expressed as oleic acid, of not more than 3.3 grams per 100 grams and the other characteristics of which correspond to those fixed for this category in the IOC standard. This designation may only be sold directly to the consumer if permitted in the country of retail sale. If not permitted, the designation of this product has to comply with the legal provisions of the country concerned.

- Virgin olive oil not fit for consumption is classed as lampante virgin olive oil, virgin olive oil which has a free acidity, expressed as oleic acid, of more than 3.3 grams per 100 grams and/or the organoleptic characteristics and other characteristics of which correspond to those fixed for this category in the IOC standard. It is intended for refining or technical use.

- Refined olive oil is the olive oil obtained from virgin olive oils by refining methods which do not lead to alterations in the initial glyceridic structure. It has a free acidity, expressed as oleic acid, of no more than 0.3 grams per 100 grams, and its other characteristics correspond to those fixed for this category in the IOC standard. This designation may only be sold directly to the consumer if permitted in the country of retail sale.

- Olive oil is the oil consisting of a blend of refined olive oil and virgin olive oils fit for consumption as they are. It has a free acidity, expressed as oleic acid, of no more than 1 gram per 100 grams, and its other characteristics correspond to those fixed for this category in the IOC standard. The country of retail sale may require a more specific designation.

- Olive pomace oil is the oil obtained by treating olive pomace with solvents or other physical treatments, to the exclusion of oils obtained by esterification processes and of any mixture with oils of other kinds. It is marketed by the following designations and definitions:

    - *Crude olive pomace* is olive pomace oil whose characteristics correspond to those fixed for this category in the IOC standard. It is intended for human consumption, or it is intended for technical use.

    - *Refined olive pomace* is the oil obtained from crude olive pomace oil by refining methods which do not lead to alterations in the initial glyceridic structure. It has a free acidity, expressed as oleic acid, of no more than 0.3 grams per 100 grams, and its other characteristics correspond to those fixed for this category in the IOC standard. This product may only be sold directly to the consumer if permitted in the country of retail sale.

    - *Olive pomace* is the oil comprising the blend of refined olive pomace oil and virgin olive oils fit for consumption as they are. It has a free acidity of no more than 1 gram per 100 grams, and its other characteristics correspond to those fixed for this category in the IOC standard. The country of retail sale may require a more specific designation.

Olive Oil Grade Descriptions from the United States International Trade Commission

- Virgin oils: oils obtained from olives that have not undergone any treatment other than washing, decanting, centrifugation, and filtration. Virgin oil is obtained during the first pressing of whole olives.
- Extra-virgin: The highest grade of virgin olive oil, which exhibits some fruitiness and is free of taste defects.
- Virgin: Oil that is fit for human consumption, has reasonably good flavor, but may exhibit taste defects.
- Lampante virgin: Virgin oil that is not fit for human consumption without further processing and contains flavor and odor defects.
- Olive oil: Oil that is made from blending virgin and refined olive oil. This oil is fit for human consumption and makes up the majority of global olive oil sales.
- Refined olive oil: Olive oil that has been refined into an edible product yet maintains the initial glyceridic structure of olive oil. The refining process heats the oil to get rid it of flavor flaws such as rancidity. Refined oil does not contain the same beneficial nutrients as virgin oil.
- Olive pomace oil: Olive pomace is the solid remains (skins, pulp, seeds, etc.) left over from the first press of olives for oil. Olive pomace oil is extracted from the pomace using chemical solvents and must be refined to be fit for human consumption. Once refined, it is mixed with virgin oils for consumption.

Olive Oil Tasting

Appreciating good olive oil requires an understanding of two essential senses: taste and smell. Tasting olive oil is like wine tasting; it is a sensory experience, an acquired taste. A newbie to wine tasting cannot differentiate between an inexpensive bottle and an excellent vintage one unless he understands how grapes from different regions picked at various harvests can influence quality. He must also be able to recognize positive attributes of the wine. The same goes for olive oil. Both contain aromatic molecules and high antioxidant polyphenols; both are rich, fragrant, and full of flavor.

Unlike other vegetable oils, olive oil must be tested for three positive attributes before it can be graded. Once you learn how to recognize the subtle but unique aromas and how to identify the different tastes, it will be less of a mystery. Laboratory analyses and official techniques are required for official tasting, but with time, you too can evaluate extra-virgin olive oil in three steps: pouring, smelling, and sipping the oil.

Virgin olive oil is the only food product that must have mandatory sensory tests before bottling. Although the chemical analysis is necessary and takes place at the same time, that alone cannot determine the flavor and aroma of the oil. Professionally trained tasters follow strict guidelines set by the International Olive Council when testing the oil for taste.

The first test is to check the acidity level of the oil. For extra-virgin olive oil, this must not be more than 0.8%. The chemical test takes place in a laboratory, not through tasting by professionals. "Acidity level" does not mean that it leaves an acid taste in the mouth. It indicates good quality, showing the oil has a low level of oleic free acid with no sensory flaws. The condition of the fruit at the time of processing has a direct influence on the acid level—a higher level shows that the fruit might be overripe, that it might have been overheated

during production, or that there was too much time between picking and processing.

Official testing usually takes place with eight to twelve professional tasters who sip different oils from numbered samples. They
judge according to three attributes: fruitiness, pungency, and bitterness. The oils are first warmed to a temperature of 26.5° C (80°
F), and then presented in little blue bottles so that the tasters aren't
influenced by color. Extra-virgin olive oil can vary in color, from
green to golden, but color does not indicate quality. The tasters
classify the oil according to flavor and the presence or absence of
defects. "Defects" refer to the negative aspects of the oil. For example, the oil could have a rancid taste because the oil is too old or it
could be made with bad olives. Pure extra-virgin olive oil has no
defects.

Tasters have to assess the properties of the oil and note the score
on the organoleptic profile sheet. After analyzing the data, the oils
are then classified into the categories of extra-virgin, virgin, and
lampante oil. In excellent oils, these characteristics of fruitiness,
pungency, and bitterness are harmoniously balanced, together with
complex aromas, flavors, and aftertastes picked up through olfactory, gustatory, and tactile sensations.

You might find yourself in a store where they invite you to taste
the oil before you buy. Just like the official tasters, you need to think
of the three attributes: fruitiness when you smell and taste the oil
and bitterness and pungency recognized by tasting.

To conduct your sensory test, first warm the container with
both hands, close your eyes, and smell the oil; this is, by far, the best
way to identify the aroma of the extra-virgin olive oil. It is easy to
understand why. Scientists say the human nose, with four hundred
olfactory sensors, is capable of detecting more than ten thousand
odors, so the nose is the best machine for detecting both pleasant
and unpleasant smells. Though we underrate our sense of smell, it

is probably the most sensitive and evocative of the senses, which we can never replace with a machine.

A good olive oil gives good aromas when you smell it. Most importantly, it should have a pleasant smell, like the olive fruit. In other words, as we inhale, it should evoke a fruity sensation. The word "fruity" is often used to describe the aroma of olive oil.

You'll hear tasters talk of two distinct types of fruity oil. They are referring to the variety and the time at which the fruit was harvested. Olives picked early in the season can be classed as fruity green. These have aromas of herbaceous plants, grass, the tomato plant, banana skin, basil, the leaf of an olive tree, artichoke, the green almond, or green olives. On the other hand, when the fruit is picked when ripe, you get more mature oil, a ripe fruitiness with warmer notes such as banana, red fruit, dried fruit, exotic fruit, apple, cocoa, and tomato.

Above all, seek out freshness; a good extra-virgin olive oil cannot smell or taste moldy, rancid, cooked, greasy, meaty, metallic, or like cardboard.

Once you've recognized the positive fruity aspect by smelling, you are ready to taste. Cup the container in your hands for a few minutes then take in a sip, holding the liquid in your mouth for a few moments, not swallowing straightaway. Rather, let the oil linger in your mouth for a while. Pay attention to mouthfeel—it's better for the oil to be crisp and clean rather than flabby, coarse, or greasy.

As you take it into your mouth, the oil reaches your body temperature of 37° C (98.6° F). Because our mouths connect with our nasal cavities at the back of the throat, aromas and flavors come together, allowing us to experience taste. Sensory scientists call this the "retronasal" sensation.

If it is a good quality olive oil, you will feel the bitterness at the back of the tongue caused by the polyphenols, the strong natural antioxidants present in the oil. The earlier the fruit is harvested, the bitterer and better it is.

Pungency, also due to healthy polyphenols, is not a taste but a stinging sensation, a chemical reaction that we detect in the throat as we swallow. Taking a good mouthful of the oil is vital, as the entire mouth cavity becomes involved in olive oil tasting, from the front of the mouth to the sides of the tongue as well as the palate support and the throat.

All extra-virgin oils should have these positive attributes; if it is very pungent and bitter, we can say the oil is robust, but if the tickle has less of a kick, then consider it a smooth oil.

To summarize, by smelling the oil, we discover the fruitiness, and by tasting, we detect the fruitiness (by retro-olfaction), bitterness, and pungency—all good characteristics of extra-virgin olive oil that describe its style and complexity. Importantly, a high concentration of bitterness and pungency prevents the fats from going rancid, thus allowing the oil to stay fresh for a longer time.

As you smell and taste, here are some points you should be looking for:

- Is the aroma pleasant? Is it mild, strong, or between the two?
- Is the oil bitter? Is the bitterness strong, medium, or mild?
- Look out for pungency, that peppery bite when you swallow. Did it make you cough?

You do not have to be an expert to taste a good olive oil; it must, above all, be pleasurable, and cooking with olive oil must be a joyful experience. Let it be a hedonistic experience.

Learn about the different varieties of olives and terroirs, the various types of fruity oils, and varying intensities and pay attention to what sensory notes emerge. This will pave the way for food and olive oil matches.

With time and practice, you'll come to detect nuances in each of these groups and even start using the same vocabulary as the experts for tasting. You'll be able to describe your olive oil sample as medium fruity green with notes of artichoke and grass. Your taste buds will detect flavors you might describe as medium bitterness and a long and persistent pungency in all the palate. One oil may remind you of June when people mow their lawns when another oil tastes strongly of freshly cut herbs. Oddly enough, freshly cut grass is one of the aromatic notes that can be found in the fruity extra-virgin olive oil.

And the more you taste, the better you become.

OLIVE OIL IN THE KITCHEN

A long time ago, the Minoans, a Bronze Age civilization, lived on the island we now know as Crete. They grew barley, grapes, and olives and, according to archeological evidence, traded their olive oil with neighboring countries. Numerous findings on the Minoan civilization show that they used urns for storing and transporting olive oil. When historians analyzed their cooking utensils, they discovered that the Minoans also cooked with olive oil. This shows just how far back the art of cooking with olive oil goes— from the third millennium to 1100 BC.

Over the years, we have discovered thousands of uses for olive oil, from health and cosmetics to household remedies and cooking, where olive oil plays an undisputed vital role today.

At one time, olive oil was limited to the elite; you could find olive oil only in the Mediterranean region or in certain luxury delicatessens. That is no longer the case. Today, we have become more curious. We want to learn more about the different flavors of olive oil, and we want to find new ways of using it in the kitchen. And, because we are more health conscious, we explore the health benefits.

Olive oil has become associated with Mediterranean cuisine, another reason it has become an essential ingredient in kitchens all over the world. Raw, cooked, fried, or as a natural preservative, olive oil has numerous uses in cooking. Cooks and chefs appreciate its wide range of flavors and aromas; they know that cooking with olive oil means fine cuisine with good flavor and aroma. What's good to know, too, is that even if we cook with olive oil, it still retains its nutritional value.

We get the best nutritional and aromatic properties of extra-virgin olive oil from newly pressed oil obtained from fruit picked green or just when the color is about to change. We want to keep those two properties, but if we increase our heating temperatures whilst cooking, we damage the natural antioxidants present in the oil. The highly prized vitamin E, for example, is one of those precious antioxidants which loses its qualities, and can even be eliminated, through natural oxidation, cooking, and repeated heating.

Drizzling and dipping olive oil over food are easy ways to take in the daily recommended olive oil without cooking or heating. Here are some popular methods of incorporating olive oil into meals:

- Add flavor and color to a dish of steamed fish or mashed potatoes with a dash of olive oil.
- Use it to provide the finishing touch to a hot dish, a favorite of food lovers.
- Drizzle a little over toasted bread with perhaps a hint of garlic.
- Drizzle some oil on goat cheese to bring out more flavors.
- Use it in a marinade. Thinly sliced beef carpaccio is a good example.
- Drizzle just a touch more olive oil on a tomato salad.
- Add it to a fresh fruit salad for a subtle, contrasting flavor.

To liven up our dishes, we can choose from a selection of olive oils flavored with different herbs, lemons, and so on; infused porcini mushrooms is a favorite with gourmets. Some mills even grind oranges or lemons along with the olives to give it an acidic flavor. And let's not forget the hot olive oil spiced with pili-pili red peppers, another favorite used for seasoning pizzas.

One renowned French chef, Mauro Colagreco, adds a creative touch to traditional cuisine by using yuzu fruit—a cross between a lemon, a mandarin, and a grapefruit—into his own brand of olive oil, "Chef's Olive Oil with Yuzu." The citrus fruit is hard to grow, expensive, and rare, but it thrives in Menton, where Colagreco lives. To make this different, subtle type of oil, they pick the fruit when it is ripe and macerate the whole fruit in extra-virgin olive oil for about a month. Mauro Colagreco uses his yuzu olive oil at all of his restaurants: The Mirazur, his elegant restaurant in Menton, one in Paris, and two in China.

Although herb-infused olive oil is gaining popularity as an easy, practical option, purists argue that these flavored varieties used in sauces and dressings distort the true flavors of olive oil. They say that olive oil already has its own complex aroma and doesn't need any other additions like garlic and basil; besides, this speeds up the unwanted oxidation and rancidity processes. The International Olive Council has a strict policy on flavored oils. They say that extra-virgin olive oils must be 100% pure and that nothing can be added, which is why flavored oils are not included in their classification of extra-virgin. These are commercially labeled as "dressings made with extra-virgin olive oil" and "flavored olive oils."

These infused olive oils, however, are great in marinades. The technique of marinating food has been around for a long time, used especially in the past to prevent food from going bad. Today, we leave meat to marinate in olive oil or wine before cooking essentially to tenderize and to add flavor.

Preserving food by marinating it was especially popular in Mediterranean countries. Marinating prevents oxidation (the reaction when food is exposed to oxygen) and hydrolysis (exposure to water). One fairly well-known Mediterranean dish, *escabeche*, is a good example of this ancient cooking method still used today. The olive oil and vinegar mixture creates a sort of seal, protecting and preserving the fish and at the same time inhibiting any contamination by microbes.

Cooking with Olive Oil

Cooking with olive oil opens up a whole new world, but one thing is sure: no matter how good the oil is, it still burns when you heat it. The chemical composition of food changes with cooking, making food easy to digest. This is a positive change, and we want it to take place. But not all changes are good. Some can be detrimental to our health, and a lot depends on the stability of the cooking oil we use.

When we cook, stew, shallow-fry, deep-fry, and sauté in extra-virgin olive oil, we lose some of the oil's nutritional and taste properties because the minor components are destroyed, especially if we use high temperatures and cook for a long time. However, all the categories of olive oil are rich in oleic acid and, therefore, high in monounsaturated fats. It is this important property that makes them more stable and makes the oil more resistant to heat. This is not the case for other vegetable oils that are rich in omega-3s.

When we talk about stability in cooking, we refer to the resistance of oil or fat to high temperatures. Olive oil is a stable oil because it has a high smoke point (the temperature at which the fat changes its chemical composition, gives off smoke, and becomes toxic). All fats, when subjected to high temperatures ($180°$ C or $356°$ F for most olive oils), undergo changes to their molecular structure. At first, they lose their organoleptic and nutritional qualities, but as the temperature rises, they deteriorate, oxidize, and finally end up being bad for our health. Virgin olive oil reaches its smoke point at $190°$ C ($374°$ F) on average, but the fresher and less acidic it is, the more stable, with the smoke point sometimes reaching $207°$ C ($404°$ F).

The smoke point is related not only to the fatty acid content but also to the presence of free fatty acids and the acidity level. That is why refined oils are more stable—the refining process that manufacturers employ eliminates these elements. The smoke point of refined sunflower oil is $232°$ C ($450°$ F), the same as refined soy oil and peanut oils. Admittedly, they have higher smoke points than olive oil, but that is because they have been refined and have undergone a chemical extraction process which has also eliminated all of their health benefits. Extra-virgin olive oil, by contrast, is a pure, natural fruit juice.

Frying is a popular method of cooking in all Mediterranean countries, regardless of religion. It consists of immersing food in oil that is already heated at a temperature of between 130° C and 180° C (226–356° F)—the ideal temperature for cooking food quickly without reaching the smoke point. (If the oil is heated beforehand, the food absorbs much less oil as it cooks.) Extra-virgin olive oil is ideal because of its composition of fatty acids and low acidity, qualities which make it more stable.

When you fry with olive oil, a crust forms around the food, providing a sort of protection envelope around the food; this means that the oil does not seep in. At the same time, it makes the food crunchy and tasty.

Frying in Olive Oil

To fry or not to fry with olive oil? This has been an ongoing subject of debate for chefs, but a new study shows that even with frying, we can still enjoy the benefits of olive oil. This nutritional discovery suggests that frying with extra-virgin olive oil improves the nutritional profile of our vegetables better than boiling them.

In 2015, Jessica del Pilar Ramírez Anaya, under the supervision of Dr. Cristina Samaniego Sánchez of the University of Granada in Spain, set out to study "phenols and the antioxidant capacity of Mediterranean vegetables prepared with extra-virgin olive oil using different domestic cooking techniques." In other words, the aim of her study was to see what happens to the natural antioxidants and phenols in vegetables when you cook them in extra-virgin olive oil.

Ramírez Anaya chose four common vegetables of the Mediterranean diet—the potato, the tomato, the aubergine (eggplant), and the pumpkin. The vegetables were cooked using three basic methods—deep-fried, sautéed, and boiled. 120 grams of each vegetable without the skin or seeds were boiled in water, boiled in a mix of water and olive oil, or fried or sautéed for ten minutes in extra-virgin olive oil.

The study was performed using good quality extra-virgin olive oil with low acidity which had been adequately stored. The frying time was limited to ten minutes and the cooking temperature to 180° C (356° F).

The study results, published in *Food Chemistry* in December 2015, showed that frying vegetables in extra-virgin olive oil improved the antioxidant content of the food much more than ordinary cooking methods. The researchers say a larger quantity of the polyphenols present in the extra-virgin olive oil was transferred to the food through frying, much more than through the other cooking methods.

According to Ramírez Anaya: "In the household conditions of the study, using extra-virgin olive oil for frying is recommendable if we wish to increase the level of monounsaturated fatty acids in the lipid profile of food and improve the polyphenol content of vegetables, which is naturally low."

We must remember, though, that deep-frying still increases the caloric density of food. Ramírez Anaya, who earned her doctorate though the study, reminds us that "that is why we insist on the recommendation to limit the consumption of fried food in our daily diet, as it is high in calories; it's also very tempting and not recommended for a modern sedentary lifestyle."

So, as frying increases the caloric density of food, a small amount of fried food is beneficial; it should just be consumed in moderation.

Food and Oil Combinations

We have to remember that there is not one good type of oil, but many. Olive oil is a fruit juice that covers a very broad aromatic palette, with different varieties; various types of fruitiness; and different intensities of fruitiness, bitterness, and spiciness. This great wealth of flavors allows for a myriad of uses and recipes and means that oils can be combined in a dish. To get more information on the organoleptic profile of an extra-virgin olive oil, we need to look at the olive variety or varieties that make up the oil. A combination of different varieties is called a "blend," whereas oil made from only one variety is called "single varietal."

There are more than 1,700 listed varieties in the world, as well as those not yet identified. As with wine, each variety is an ensemble of unique qualities that are expressed physically through the shape of the leaves, the fruit, the color, the chemical composition of the olive, and all the particularities that give it its own unique sensory profile. Some varieties produce a soft and pure juice, while others yield intense fruity green oil, even though they are harvested over the same period and from the same place. The variety is widely responsible for this organoleptic profile.

These days, you'll find the olive variety displayed prominently on the label; this information is helpful to the consumer looking to cook or season a dish. Here are some examples:

- If you need soft and delicate oil for a dessert, it is best to choose a Spanish Arbequina or a Portuguese Arbosana.
- A spicy Coratina is ideal for an oven-baked pizza.
- A French Négrette is great on mashed potatoes.
- A Koroneiki works well on a Greek salad.

Ideally, a cook should have oils of different varieties on hand to enhance each dish. This aspect of cooking has, up until now, received little attention, but it offers a wealth of opportunities. We should feel free to experiment with contrasting flavors by adding an intense fruity green olive oil to vanilla ice cream, for example, or we could combine complementary aromas such as tomato-flavored oil with a salad of tomato, mozzarella, and basil. We could also try using mild oil on a very delicate dish or on food that doesn't require intense flavors, such as desserts or mayonnaise.

Matching oils to dishes is a new discipline, so no cookbooks have yet been written on the subject. However, here are a few fundamental and accepted rules:

- Good-quality oils improve the taste of all food, whether served hot or cold.
- The de-sugaring quality of olive oil allows us to prepare desserts that don't feel fatty or sugary.
- The bitterness of olive oil normally does not go well with a dish that already has a bitter flavor (like meat) as it further accentuates the taste, but with some foods, it's an amazing pairing (as in the case of chocolate with a strong Picual).
- Extra-virgin olive oil enhances flavors and aromas, intensifying our sensory perception.

As we mentioned before, although olive oil is a healthy fat, it is a fat nevertheless and very high in calories. Like all vegetable oils, olive oil is a high-energy food, providing nine kilocalories per gram—more than butter, which provides 7.5 kilocalories per gram. We should, therefore, consume it in moderation if we wish to stay in shape and follow the recommendations of the World Health Organization. They tell us, broadly speaking, to consume less saturated fat, trans-fatty acids, free sugars, and salt and to eat more fruit, vegetables, whole-grain cereals, and nuts.

The golden rules are to eat fresh and seasonal food and to combine oils but always with a preference for omega-9 and raw omega-3 oils—always in small quantities. Equally important: we should go for quality rather than quantity, keep active, and take our time when cooking. In short, follow the fundamental principles of Mediterranean cuisine.

Recipes We Love

These are some of our favorite recipes, ones that we have made and tried; they're not taken from cookbooks but come from our friends and family. We even have one from Dr. Amal Kaddoumi (Wonder 5: Olive Oil Slows Alzheimer's Disease).

BEAUTIFUL HEALTHY MAYONNAISE

From Cécile

Did you know that most shop-bought mayonnaise is full of bad fats? Making your own mayonnaise is so easy and so much better for your health, especially if you use extra-virgin olive oil (EVOO) and a free-range egg. Mayonnaise will keep for about a week if you store it in a sterilized jar in the fridge. And once you've tasted it, you won't want store-bought mayonnaise again. It's okay to be nervous the first time you make your own mayonnaise, but be patient; it's worth it.

1 free-range egg yolk	Salt and pepper
1 tablespoon vinegar (15 milliliters)	1 cup EVOO (1/4 liter or 240
1 heaping teaspoon mustard	milliliters)

In a deep bowl, mix the egg yolk, vinegar, and mustard. Add salt and pepper.

Add a little olive oil in a steady stream, mixing with a whisk until the mixture has thickened. Some use a fork, but you could use a whisk or an electric beater, starting with a little oil in the beginning and beating until the mixture thickens then adding more oil gradually. Taste it, and if you like it and are feeling adventurous, you might want to add a clove of garlic, some fresh herbs, or a bit more salt and pepper.

Shish Kebab Lamb

From Alice

This is one of my favorite recipes. Lamb marinated this way is wickedly delicious and so easy to prepare. What's good is that you can do most of it the night before. You can also double the proportions for a crowd.

4 tablespoons honey (60 milliliters)

2 pounds lamb (1 kilogram)

Juice of 1 lemon

2 tablespoons oyster sauce (30 milliliters)

3 tablespoons EVOO (45 milliliters)

1 tablespoon seasoning salt (15 milliliters)

2 tablespoons Worcestershire sauce (30 milliliters)

3 tablespoons Lea & Perrins sauce (45 milliliters)

1 tablespoon garlic powder (15 milliliters)

1 small pineapple, cut into bite-size pieces

Microwave the honey for a minute or two until it has melted. Allow to cool. Prepare a marinade of oyster sauce, olive oil, seasoning salt, Worcestershire sauce, Lea & Perrins sauce, garlic powder, and the honey.

Cut the lamb into bite-sized pieces, soak in lemon juice for about 5 minutes, then rinse with cold water and pat dry.

Season the lamb with the marinade and refrigerate overnight.

The following day, once the meat has had time to become tender, heat the barbecue. Drain the marinade from the meat and set aside. On skewers, place lamb and pineapple chunks alternately.

Place the skewers on the barbecue. Cook for about 20–25 minutes or until the lamb is cooked, turning and basting with the marinade from time to time.

This lamb goes well with garlic mashed potatoes.

TAPENADE

From Cécile

I asked Anne-Laure Meunier, French nutritionist (see page 15, "Understanding Fats"), what her favorite recipe was from olives and olive oil. Without hesitating and with a broad smile, she said, "La tapenade!" Tapenade is a Provençal favorite, made with green olives, black olives, or both! It's perfect for picnics and can be served with drinks, at tapas parties, and even as an hors d'oeuvre. Serve it with tiny toasted bread slices or crackers. Traditionally, it is made using a mortar and pestle, but you can get equally good results using a food processor.

1 cup black pitted and minced olives (180 grams)	1 tablespoon capers (14 grams)
	1 garlic clove
1 cup green pitted and minced olives (180 grams)	1 anchovy fillet
	1/4 cup EVOO(60 milliliters)

Mix all the ingredients together to form a smooth paste or make it coarse and rustic. Once made, put it in the fridge a few minutes before serving.

● Extras

Once you create your paste, try adding one or two of these ingredients: fresh chopped parsley, basil, oregano, thyme, or even a bit of lemon juice.

Adding homemade tapenade to baked fish will make it moist and delicious. You can use it as a stuffing, spread it on top of the fish before you put it in the oven, or just spread the tapenade on top of fish fillets, roll them up, and secure with toothpicks. Bake the fish as you would normally.

SALMON FILLETS COOKED NADIA'S WAY

From Alice

This recipe comes from my friend and good neighbor Nadia. This is her very own recipe—a warm, elegant, yet simple starter for chilly days. Fish, ginger, and olive oil can only be healthy and full of goodness, but when I tried to make this dish for the first time, I ran into some difficulties when frying the fillet. I have included some advice to make frying easier.

As salmon is such a tender fish; it is important not to let it stick to the pan when pan-frying. Bear in mind that you want to lift the fillets without tearing them, so make sure that the pan is hot enough, that the fillets are not crowded, and that you have enough oil. Remember, too, that salmon has a tendency to curl up as you fry, so use a flexible metal spatula to hold it firmly in place as you cook the bottom and use the spatula also for flipping over. I preheated the pan then reduced the temperature.

Also, make sure your guests are sitting, ready and waiting, for this starter. This dish needs to be served warm.

3 tablespoons EVOO for the vinaigrette (45 milliliters)
Extra olive oil for frying
Juice of 1 lime
Salt and freshly ground pepper
4 salmon fillets, about 120 grams
each

A mix of mesclun and rocket salad
A stick of fresh ginger, about 1
centimeter long
4 cooked prawns
Some spring onions (cleaned and
chopped finely)

Make a vinaigrette using 3 tablespoons olive oil, lime juice, salt, and pepper and set aside.

Prepare the pan and cook the salmon in the remaining oil. First, cook skin side down for 5 minutes. Then flip over and cook the other side for about 3 minutes. They should retain their texture and pink color.

Wrap the fillets in some aluminum foil to keep them warm while you prepare the plates.

Prepare the serving dishes, starting with the salad then placing the fillets in the middle. Finely grate the ginger over the salmon. Decorate with the prawns and spring onions, and then cover it all with the vinaigrette before serving.

Manakish

From Dr. Amal Kaddoumi

This is a flatbread from the Eastern Mediterranean region. The dough, Amal says, can be basic pizza dough, either homemade or store bought.

1 package pre-made pizza dough   1 tablespoon za'atar (roasted
3 tablespoons EVOO   thyme)

Preheat oven to 350° F (177° C) or according to package directions. Spread the dough onto a lightly floured work surface and gently knead one or two times before using. Use your hands to flatten the dough and round the edges. Top the dough with olive oil (a generous amount!). Sprinkle with za'atar and bake until just crisp.

MADELEINES OR SHELL-SHAPED COOKIES

From Cécile

This one comes from Lola, my Spanish mother-in-law. She makes these every week and serves them for breakfast or at coffee time. I especially like these because it's wonderful to be able to replace butter with olive oil in a dessert and it's so simple to put together. Makes 30 madeleine cookies.

3 eggs

1/2 teaspoon salt

1 1/4 cups sugar (250 grams)

1 cup EVOO (1/4 liter or 240 milliliters)

8 ounces milk

Zest of 1 lemon

2 teaspoons baking powder (1.5 grams)

2 1/2 cups flour (300 grams)

30 paper liners

Optional: chocolate or chocolate chips

Preheat oven to 355° F (180° C).

Separate the eggs. Put the whites and a pinch of salt in a bowl. Beat the whites until they are stiff and then add the yolks. Add the sugar, oil, milk, lemon zest, baking powder, and flour. Put these ingredients in slowly and stir after each addition.

Using a teaspoon measurer, half fill each paper cup. Sprinkle each madeleine with a little sugar and put them in the preheated oven. Don't open the door until the madeleines are golden brown (about 5–10 minutes). Remove them when they are brown and allow them to cool. They are ready! Lola warns that these madeleines bake very quickly, so you do need to be careful if your oven is a fast one like hers.

If you like chocolate, why not fill the cookies with melted chocolate or chocolate chips? Just add a teaspoon of melted chocolate as you're filling the paper cups or add the chocolate chips at the same time as you sprinkle the sugar before baking.

PROVENÇAL-STYLE YOGURT CAKE WITH QUINCE

From Alice

One of the first things children learn to make in France is a yogurt cake. It's easy because they don't have to measure anything. All they need is a pot of yogurt—they empty it, rinse it, dry it, and use it to measure the rest of the ingredients.

This jazzed-up variation incorporates ground almonds and quince, a recipe that my good friend Madeleine from Cooking in Provence *taught in her cooking class. The "pot" refers to a pot of yogurt. In France, our pots of yogurt contain 250 grams, but the recipe works with any size. You might just have to watch the baking powder quantity if your pots of yogurt are over 250 grams.*

1 quince	Zest of 1 lemon
1 pot sugar	2 pots flour
4 eggs	3/4 teaspoon baking powder
2 pots plain yogurt	2 pots ground almonds
1 pot EVOO	

Preheat oven to 355° F (180°C).

Core the quince, then place it in a saucepan with a spoonful of sugar and cover with water. Bring to a boil and cook uncovered until tender.

In a large mixing bowl, whisk the eggs and sugar until the mixture is quite pale. Stir in the yogurt, olive oil, and lemon zest until all the ingredients are fully incorporated. Add the flour, baking powder, and almonds.

Grease a baking tin and pour in the batter. Arrange the quince on top.

Bake for about 45 minutes, checking the center of the cake with a fork to make sure that the cake is cooked.

Remove the cake from the oven, but let cool for 10 minutes or so before removing from the cake tin.

BAKED ARTICHOKE

From Cécile

I love this recipe because it's so simple yet nutritious and delicious! If you plan to serve it as a main course, I recommend three small artichokes per person. As a starter, one artichoke per person will be enough. I learned this recipe in Barcelona, where they have a lot of artichoke fields and just as many ways to cook it.

4 artichokes	a robust one (60–90 milliliters)
Salt and pepper, to taste	Extra ingredients: garlic, paprika,
4–6 tablespoons EVOO, preferably	ham or bacon

Preheat oven to 355° F (180°C).

Cut away any excess stems, then cut the artichokes in half from top to bottom, making sure you remove any hair that you sometimes get in the middle of an artichoke. Rinse well and place an oven-proof dish (leaves facing down). Sprinkle with salt and pepper and drizzle with olive oil.

Bake the artichokes for 30 minutes. You will know they're cooked when the first leaves become slightly charred. When the artichokes are cooked, remove them, put in a serving dish, and drizzle with a little more olive oil (and any optional toppings). Serve hot.

During the summer, you can follow the same recipe but cook them on a barbecue. Yum!

Provençal Tomatoes

From Alice

Simple, easy-to-make Provençal tomatoes are perfect with grilled steak or as a starter. I particularly love this recipe; it's one of my standby meals and one I can make almost with my eyes closed. It always goes down well with family, friends, and neighbors who drop in for drinks and get invited to an impromptu dinner. Just double the quantities if you expect a crowd.

4 ripe tomatoes
2 cloves crushed garlic
1 tablespoon fresh parsley (15 milliliters)

1 tablespoon fresh thyme (15 milliliters)
2 tablespoons bread crumbs (30 mililiters)
EVOO for sprinkling over

Preheat oven to 400° F (200° C).

Cut the tomatoes in half; remove the seeds and flesh with a spoon and sprinkle with salt. Turn tomatoes upside down to drain for 10 minutes. When drained, place tomatoes in a gratin dish.

Mix the garlic, parsley, and thyme in a bowl. Fill each of the tomatoes with the mixture, top with breadcrumbs, sprinkle with olive oil, and bake for about 20 minutes.

OLIVE OIL QUIZ

Are you an olive oil expert? This simple quiz will test your knowledge. Check the answers at the end to see how well you did.

1. WHAT IS THE PROPORTION OF LIPIDS IN EXTRA-VIRGIN OLIVE OIL?

    a. Around 75%
    b. Around 100%
    c. Around 98%–99%

2. HOW MANY KILOGRAMS OF OLIVES DO YOU NEED TO PRODUCE ONE LITER OF EXTRA-VIRGIN OLIVE OIL?

    a. Between 4 and 10 kilograms
    b. Less than 4 kilograms
    c. Between 10 and 15 kilograms

3. WHICH COUNTRY IS THE BIGGEST PRODUCER OF OLIVES?

    a. Greece
    b. Spain
    c. Italy

4. HOW MANY TABLESPOONS OF EXTRA-VIRGIN OLIVE OIL DO THE EXPERTS RECOMMEND YOU SHOULD TAKE EVERY DAY TO GET THE FULL BENEFIT OF OLEOCANTHAL?

    a. 1 tablespoon
    b. 3 tablespoons
    c. 6 tablespoons

5. WHICH OF THESE STATEMENTS ARE TRUE? (HINT: THERE ARE TWO.)

    a.   Olive oil contains vitamin E
    b.   Olive oil contains fluoride
    c.   Olive oil contains squalene
    d.   Olive oil contains caffeine

6. "BITTERNESS" AND "PUNGENCY" ARE TERMS USED TO DESCRIBE EXTRA-VIRGIN OLIVE OIL, BUT WHAT ARE THEY?

    a.   They are defects
    b.   They are the effects of high acid content
    c.   They are two positive attributes

7. WHY SHOULD YOUR BOTTLE OF EXTRA VIRGIN BE OPAQUE?

    a.   To see the label and the nutritional value better
    b.   Because color isn't a characteristic of quality
    c.   To protect the oil from the light

8. WHICH IS THE BEST PLACE TO STORE OLIVE OIL?

    a.   Under the sink
    b.   In a refrigerator under 7° C (45° F)
    c.   Out of the light and between 15°C and 20° C (59° F and 68° F)

9. WHICH OF THE FOLLOWING STATEMENTS IS TRUE WHEN WE TALK ABOUT TABLE OLIVES?

    a.   They can be eaten directly from the tree
    b.   They do not contain oil
    c.   Some varieties are better for table olives, others for oil, and some for both

10. HYDROXYTYROSOL IS . . .

    a.   A phenolic component
    b.   A fertilizer
    c.   Strong bacteria which kills olive trees

11. WHICH OF THE FOLLOWING DESCRIBES OLIVE OIL?

a. Has a high level of oleic acid
b. Has a high level of palmitic acid
c. Has a high level of free fatty acid

12. WHAT DOES "COLD" MEAN IN "FIRST COLD PRESS"?

a. The cold chain must not be interrupted while processing the oil
b. To comply with regulations, the temperature must be less than 27° C (81° F) during the olive paste kneading
c. Producers wait until the winter to begin harvesting and processing olives

13. WHICH OF THESE OIL CROPS IS THE MOST PRODUCED OIL IN THE WORLD?

a. Soybeans
b. Rapeseed
c. Palm kernels

14. HOW LONG CAN YOU KEEP YOUR BOTTLE OF OLIVE OIL?

a. Olive oil is like wine; the longer you keep it, the better
b. Around two or three years
c. Around one year

15. OLEOCANTHAL IS ONE OF THE MOST IMPORTANT COMPONENTS IN EXTRA-VIRGIN OLIVE OIL. WHICH OF THESE IS THE BEST METHOD OF CHECKING THE LEVEL OF OLEOCANTHAL IN THE BOTTLE?

a. Read the label; it will state the percentage clearly
b. Take a sip and see if you get a sting at the back of your throat
c. Smell it; it will have a strong but sweet smell

16. SOME FATTY ACIDS ARE GOOD FOR OUR HEALTH, BUT WHICH FATTY OIL SHOULD YOU NOT USE FOR FRYING AND COOKING?

    a.   Oils rich in omega-9 acids
    b.   Oils rich in omega-3 acids
    c.   Oils rich in omega-6 acids

17. WHICH OF THESE STATEMENTS IS CORRECT?

    a.   Olive oil contains a small amount of calcium
    b.   Olive oil does not contain any calcium
    c.   Olive oil contains a lot of calcium

18. WHAT IS THE MARKET SHARE OF OLIVE OIL IN THE GLOBAL EDIBLE OIL MARKET?

    a.   1%
    b.   3%
    c.   10%

19. WHAT HAPPENS WHEN A VEGETABLE OIL REACHES ITS SMOKE POINT?

    a.   It gives off a pleasant aroma
    b.   The oil is hot enough and ready for frying foods
    c.   The oil has been destroyed and has become toxic to our health

20. WHY DOES OLIVE OIL HAVE GOOD STABILITY FOR FRYING OR COOKING?

    a.   It is composed mostly of monounsaturated fats
    b.   It is composed mainly of saturated fatty acids
    c.   It is a natural juice that has not been refined

21. HOW DO WE GET THE MOST NUTRITIONAL AND AROMATIC QUALITIES OUT OF EXTRA-VIRGIN OLIVE OIL?

    a.   By frying
    b.   Having it raw
    c.   *En papillote*

22. What does "extra-virgin olive oil matching" mean?

d.   It is something that the renowned Spanish chef Ferran Adrià
     invented
e.   It is a new discipline
a.   It is a discipline that has disappeared

23. The sensorial analysis test for olive oil . . .

a.   Is compulsory
b.   Is one of two choices: chemical analysis or sensorial analysis
c.   Is not necessary

24. When choosing olive oil, what is the first thing you must look for?

a.   The category it belongs to
b.   The deadline for optimal consumption
c.   Where the olives come from

25. Which category below can be purchased commercially?

a.   Pure olive oil
b.   Olive pomace oil
c.   Lampante olive oil

Answers

Here are the answers to the questions. If you got 20 correct answers, then you are an expert on olive oil matters. If you got between 15 and 19 right answers, it shows you have a reasonably good knowledge.

1. Extra-virgin olive oil is characterized by a range of minor components (total: 0.5–1.5%) and a lipids portion of between 98–99%.

2. This can vary. It depends mainly on the olives; different types of olives produce different yields. In California, for example, producers need 4–10 kilograms of olives of the popular Manzanillo and Mission varieties to produce 1 liter of oil. Other contributing factors are the size of the tree, the age, how it is watered, and the climatic conditions.

3. Currently, Spain is the biggest olive oil–producing country in the world, averaging around 1,536,600 tons annually and accounting for 45% of the total world production. Italy comes second, producing around 450,000 tons annually, and in third place is Greece, with 230,000 tons per year.

4. Dr. Breslin, who conducted research on oleocanthal and cancer cells, thinks we should have 50 milliliters of extra-virgin olive oil per day, the equivalent of 3–4 tablespoons. Dr. Kaddoumi, who did studies on Alzheimer's, recommends the same amount. It might seem like a high fat content, but the majority of the fat is monounsaturated fat—healthy dietary fat—as opposed to saturated fat.

5. Two of these statements are correct. Olive oil contains the vital antioxidant vitamin E. Olive oil also contains squalene. Recent studies show that the squalene content in olive oil has a cancer risk–reducing effect.

6. Bitterness, pungency, and fruitiness are the three positive attributes you should look for when tasting olive oil. Bitterness is the taste you feel on the back of the tongue, and pungency is the sensation at the back of the throat. Bitterness and pungency are due to the phenolic compounds present in extra-virgin olive oil. For the consumer, this means that the olive oil is fresh and full of antioxidants.

7. Extra-virgin olive oil is very sensitive to photo-oxidation caused by light, oxygen, and heat. Glass bottles and opaque packaging are better than transparent and plastic bottles. Also, proper storage conditions will help maintain the nutritional and sensorial properties of extra-virgin olive oil much longer.

8. Extra-virgin olive oil is very sensitive to photo-oxidation caused by light, oxygen, and heat. To limit oxidation and to conserve your extra-virgin olive oil, you should keep it at a temperature between 15° C and 20° C (59° F and 68° F). (Most wine cellars meet these conditions.) You should not store extra-virgin olive oil under the sink, because the humidity will affect the flavor.

9. The correct answer is "Some varieties are better for table olives, other for oil, and some for both." It all depends on the variety of olives and the quantity of oil or pulp. In most cases, you can't eat olives directly from the tree, because they are much too bitter; they have to be treated to remove the bitterness before you add them to your salads. When they're picked young, you get green olives; when they're picked at full maturity, you get black olives.

10. Hydroxytyrosol is a polyphenol, a powerful antioxidant contained in the olive leaf and olive oil. Concentration can vary depending on the variety, oil producing techniques, how ripe the fruit was at picking, storage before extracting the oil, and the method used for extraction.

11. Olive oil is characterized by a high level of oleic acid; between 55% and 83%. Cultivars vary, but the oil will contain 8%–20% of palmitic acid and 4%–21% of linoleic acid. Its oxidative stability is linked to the fatty acid composition of the oil, particularly the high level of oleic acid. This high level of oleic acid allows olive oil to be classed as a monounsaturated fatty acid.

12. The first option is the correct answer—the cold chain must not be interrupted during the entire process. This means that, following regulations, the olives are kept at less than 27° C (80° F) during processing so as to retain the nutrients and lessen the degradation of the oil. Interestingly, there is a difference between cold extraction and cold pressing. Regulations in Europe stipulate that when a centrifuge, the modern method of extraction for large quantities, is used, the label must say "cold extracted," while only a physically pressed olive oil may be marked as "cold pressed." In many parts of the world, you'll see "cold pressed" on the label even if the producers used centrifugal extraction.

13. The outlook for the market season 2015/2016 shows global soybean production yield at 318 million tons followed by rapeseed with 64.3 tons and palm kernels at 15.8 tons.

14. The "use by" date usually guarantees the best organoleptic properties of the olive oil, around one year, but it depends on the variety (some can be kept more than two years), the phenolic compounds, and how it's stored. For example, a transparent bottle in a supermarket can suffer photo-oxidation and last less than one year. Once the bottle is opened, it's best to use it up within three months.

15. The sting at the back of the throat tells us how much oleocanthal is in the oil. Gary Beauchamp, who discovered oleocanthal, accidentally stumbled upon the similarities between ibuprofen and olive oil when he tasted olive oil for the first time.

16. Both omega-3 and -9 are polyunsaturated acids. Our bodies do not produce omega-3s: you find them in some vegetable oils (flax, hemp, rapeseed, nut) and in foods like oily fish, hazelnuts, oysters, mussels, almonds, and flaxseed. Although omega-3s are essential for our health, for proper functioning of our brain and heart, there is one downside: oils containing omega-3 acids do not do well with high temperatures and become toxic. It's best to have them raw.

17. Olive oil contains a small amount of calcium—only 1 milligram per 100 grams of oil.

18. The olive oil market accounts for less than 3% of the world edible oil market.

19. When you heat oil too much and it gives off smoke, it has reached its smoke point. Smoke point is the temperature at which the oil starts breaking down, turns black, and forms smoke. It is an indication of the stability of the oil. You need to be aware of the smoke points of various fats because fat is no longer considered healthy for consumption after it has exceeded its smoke point and has begun to break down. From this critical temperature, the oil produces highly toxic and carcinogenic compounds such as benzopyrene or acrolein.

Pan frying can be done at varying temperatures, ranging from about 50° C (122° F) for the mildest cooking up to 150° C (302° F) and sometimes more. We suggest not exceeding 200° C (392° F). The ideal temperature for a good fry is 190° C (374° F).

Not all oils are the same. They have different chemical compositions and different smoke points. Oils rich in polyunsaturated fatty acids with omega-3s are very sensitive to cooking and are best used for raw preparation. Extra-virgin olive oils with low acidity have a relatively high smoke point (190° C) due to their composition rich in monounsaturated fats. Refined oils (with the impurities removed) tend to have higher smoke points.

20. Olive oil is rich in monounsaturated fatty acids, the type of fatty acid that is considered stable for cooking. Its smoke point is somewhat elevated compared to other fats. Virgin olive oils must be of the best quality, as moisture and fatty acids reduce stability. Refined olive oils are more stable in cooking but must not exceed 220° C (428° F).

Here are the relevant smoke points:

- Extra-virgin: 190° C (374° F)
- Virgin: 216° C (421° F)
- Pomace: 238° C (460° F)
- Extra-light: 242° C (468° F)

Remember that repeated use of the oil reduces its stability. Oil should be filtered after each use to remove all excess particles. This should be done once the oil has become cold. It is generally advisable to renew the oil completely after ten frying sessions.

21. Although extra-virgin olive oil has good cooking stability, it is best taken raw to get the maximum health benefits and enjoy its wide aromatic range. Olive oil must be of the highest quality extra-virgin—and its deadline for optimal use must be respected (indicated on the label).

22. It means pairing food with olive oil, a new discipline in the culinary world.

Successful food matches in the kitchen depend upon the variety of the oils, the typical characteristics, and the type of fruitiness of the oil that will accompany the dishes. Although challenging, choosing the right olive oil for the right dish is becoming more and more popular in the kitchen, but there's no cookbook to teach it. Using extra-virgin olive oil allows the chef to develop new flavors and offers spectacular aromas for a hot main course dish as well as in desserts. This cooking art has undoubtedly a good future ahead!

23. It depends on the country where the olive oil is made and sold, but for the IOC members countries—98% of the world's production—both the chemical analysis and the sensorial analysis are compulsory. You cannot have one and not the other. Virgin olive oil is the only food product that needs a compulsory sensorial analysis before bottling.

The sensorial analysis is a real measuring tool. The human nose is the most accurate tool for detecting a sensory defect and level of palatability. At the official tasting of virgin olive oils, between eight and twelve trained experts test the samples and classify them according to presence or absence of sensory defects. These trainers have followed the IOC training course in designated laboratories. Extra-virgin olive oil cannot have any sensory defect and must have a certain fruitiness.

24. The commercial category is the first thing that you should look for when choosing or buying olive oil. You should choose an extra-virgin olive oil so as to have the best quality in terms of both taste and nutrition. Optimal consumption date and place of harvest or bottling of the oil are necessary information, but that does not guarantee that the oil comes exclusively from olives. Also, the oil might not have been cold extracted or stored in the best conditions to avoid damage.

25. You can buy olive pomace oil commercially.

When the oil is first pressed, you get leftovers from the extraction. It consists of skin, olive pits, and pulp. This paste is called the pomace of the oil. To this pomace are added chemical solvents like hexane or some very high heat, processes to get the last of the remaining oil. This is refined pomace oil. Olive pomace oil is a combination of this refined oil, virgin oil, and/or extra-virgin oil. Olive pomace oil is also used in the manufacture of soap.

Lampante oil is oil that has a high acidity level of above 3.3%. It needs to be refined before it can be used. Then it is mixed with virgin olive oil or extra virgin and called "olive oil."

Pure olive oil is a marketing name to create confusion for consumers. It is not legal to sell olive oil under this category. Pure olive oil is, in fact, lampante olive oil refined and assembled with some virgin olive oil or extra virgin. It is no longer a natural product but an industrial one.

GLOSSARY

ACIDITY

Acidity tells us about the quality of the oil; it shows how much care was taken from the time the fruit started blossoming right up to when it was ready for bottling. Acidity is a chemical parameter measured in the chemical analysis to determine the oleic acid content per 100 grams of oil. A low acidity level indicates freshness and high-quality oil. It shows that the manufacturing process was carried out under optimum conditions with a very short time between harvesting and extraction. It also indicates that processing took place using natural or mechanical methods, without any chemical additives. A high acidity level, on the other hand, is not desirable. It could mean that the oil is rancid, that the fruit was infested with fly disease or suffered fungal disease (Gloeosporium and Macrophoma are two examples), or that there was considerable time between the harvesting and extraction of the oil.

This parameter not only provides information on the degradation of the fatty acids in the oil but, more importantly for IOC standards, determines the category or grade of the olive oil. According to IOC, the oil can be classified into one of three categories:

- Extra-virgin olive oil must not have an acidity level of more than 0.8 grams of oleic acid per 100 grams.

- Virgin olive oil must not have an acidity level of more than 2 grams per 100 grams.
- Lampante virgin olive oil must not exceed 3.3 grams per 100 grams.

Acidity has no taste and has nothing to do with the acid flavor that you can feel on the tongue as with eating lemons. It is a chemical parameter measured in the laboratory; it cannot be evaluated in sensory analysis.

ANTIOXIDANTS

Although oxygen is essential for life, some molecules present in the air are directly involved in the aging process and cell damage. These molecules are called "free radicals," and they cause what is known as "oxidative stress." Some foods can help us to counteract their negative effects.

Minor components present in virgin olive oil, such as tocopherols (vitamin E) and some polyphenols (phenolic compounds), are nutritionally essential as well as significant for oil stability when cooking and for storage. The more antioxidants oil contains, the more stable it is over time.

The quantity of antioxidants is determined by several factors. The quality of the fruit before oil extraction, the extraction method, the maturity stage of the fruit, and the type of farming (rain, land, or irrigated) as well as the variety of the olive tree are all factors that determine the presence and intensity of these antioxidants.

AROMA

Aroma refers to the volatile compounds perceived by the olfactory sense. Olive oil has a broad range of aromas, each variety with its own characteristic scent. This sensation is known as the "fruitiness" of the olive oil. The aromatic profile of oil and its flavor intensity depends on the quality, olive variety, and ripeness of the fruit when harvested. One feature of extra-virgin olive oil is the presence and complexity of these aromas. By smelling, we pick up various aromas such as those found in vegetables, flowers, fruit, or spices. There are two types of fruity aromas. The first is a fruity green, which may be perceived as green grass, olive leaf, artichoke, or green olives picked at the beginning of the harvest. The second aroma, from ripe fruit, has olfactory notes that remind us of nuts, exotic fruits or berries, bananas, or apples. A harvested olive starts in a green fruit aroma which, over time, changes to ripe notes, while an olive harvested later directly gives a ripe fruit aroma.

The variety of olive is the main factor that determines the aroma of the oil. Olive oil aroma should be pleasant to the nose and have a fresh fruit scent. However, these flavors can also be unpleasant. The main defects of olive oil are musty, wet, winey, rancid, and metallic aromas, which can be due to fruit ripening, a fatty acid oxidation, or prolonged storage of olives before the extraction of the oil.

BASIC TASTES

Our sense of taste starts in the mouth. The tongue and taste buds are the fundamental instruments that allow us to perceive our sense of taste. There are four major flavors or tastes: sweet (e.g., banana), sour (lemon), salty (cheese, charcuterie, seafood), and bitter (endives, raw artichoke). A fifth flavor was discovered by the Japanese: umami (う ま み), or "tasty" in Japanese. This flavor is produced by amino acids present in protein-heavy foods like meats.

The appetite for sweet is innate in humans and also in mammals. For a feeding infant, the sucking action is related to the recognition of a sweet flavor. The taste buds on either side of our tongue allow us to experience saltiness, the presence of sodium ions. Acid generates displeasure, the bitter taste. Bitterness results in real repulsion, the taste similar to a natural form of protection, because poisons are usually bitter.

Our sense of smell allows us to perceive aromas, olfactory notes, and odors (direct and retronasal) and determine the fruitiness in extra-virgin olive oil.

Bitterness is perceived with the tongue and taste buds, whereas spiciness or pungency are tactile sensations instead of flavors.

BITTERNESS

Bitterness is one of the five basic tastes, specifically felt on the back of the tongue when tasting olive oil. Bitterness, together with fruitiness and pungency, shows quality in olive oil. It shows that the oil was produced from healthy fruit at the optimum moment of maturity and in the best condition so as not to alter the oil.

As the oil matures, it loses its bitterness; it can even disappear. The sooner the olives are picked, the more pronounced the bitterness.

FILTRATION

Filtration refers to the removal of sediment in the oil after production. It is a mixture of olive pits, pulp, and skin. Filtration extends the shelf life of the olive oil.

FIRST COLD PRESS

A method in which the components are pressed at the lowest possible temperature to extract a part of the oil they contain. This pressing preserves the oil nutrients (vitamins, tocopherols, essential fatty acids, pigments, etc.) and the aromas. Olive pomace oil comes from the second pressing of the olive paste.

Pressure

Applying pressure used to be the main means of obtaining olive oil. These devices, which separate the oil and paste, are gradually being replaced by continuous and centrifugal systems, which allow better temperature and hygiene control.

Cold Press

Cold oil extraction processes refer to manufacturing olive oil without using heat. Under EU rules, extraction processes should be kept below 27° C (80° F). (For other vegetable oils, keep below 50° C [122° F]).

FLAVOR

This is the combination of olfactory, gustatory, and tactile sensations perceived during an olive oil tasting. This is how we can evaluate the sensory appreciation of the oil. The most volatile compounds are detected first, and then, by keeping the oil in the mouth a while longer, we pick up the less volatile compounds.

MINOR COMPONENTS

Extra-virgin olive oil consists of 99% fatty acids, and the remaining 1% includes the minor components. This designation can be imprecise and confusing, since this proportion confers crucial organoleptic and compositional characteristics to the oil. Minor components can range between 1%–2% of the oil, and they include natural antioxidants, pigments that give the color to the oil (from a golden yellow to a deep green), vitamins, and volatile components responsible for the aroma and fruitiness of the olive oil.

With an entirely mechanical extraction process, rigorous temperature control, and monitoring of the developmental stages of the fruit from the tree to the table, virgin olive oil keeps many of these substances, antioxidants, and flavorings that enhance its sensory and nutritional value. Only virgin olive oil with the "extra" mention guarantees that the minor components will be intact up to the deadline of optimal consumption and will have a beneficial effect on our health and palate.

OLEIC ACID

Olive oil comprises around 99% fats. The remaining 1% are minor components. The fats of olive oil are composed of triglycerides, comprising different kinds of fatty acids. Fatty acid composition is different and unique for each vegetable oil. Oleic acid is the primary source of monounsaturated fatty acids or omega-9s. Olive oil is mainly composed of oleic acid oil, and that is the reason we say it is monounsaturated oil.

The name comes from the Roman *oleum*, which means "oil," and composes 55%–80% of the fatty acids of olive oil. We can find oleic acid in many animal or vegetable species, such as walnut, hazelnut, avocado, sesame, peanut, rapeseed oil, duck fat, mutton, and beef.

Monounsaturated fatty acids have a beneficial effect on cholesterol, lowering the "bad" cholesterol without affecting the "good" cholesterol.

OLEOCANTHAL

(See "Pungency")

OLEUROPEIN

Oleuropein is one of the main phenolic compounds, a powerful antioxidant that you find in the olive leaf, the olive tree, and olive oil. You can find it in argan oil as well. This is what gives extra-virgin olive oil that pungent, bitter taste.

Besides the many health benefits of phenolic compounds, oleuropein also prevents the premature oxidation of the oil.

OLIVE OIL

Olive oil is the fat obtained from the fruit of the olive tree (Olea europaea L.), the olive. Only olive oils that include "virgin" are exclusively obtained by mechanical or physical extraction processes. The oil will be assigned to a category once it has passed the chemical and sensory analyses. Only then can it be bottled.

Extra-Virgin Olive Oil

An extra-virgin olive oil has no sensory defects, with a fruitiness greater than or equal to 0 and less than 0.8% acidity.

Virgin Olive Oil

A virgin olive oil has a fruitiness greater than or equal to 0, a sensory evaluation of the defect below 2.5 (score from 0 to 10, 10 being the maximum intensity of defect), and an acidity between 0.8% and 2%.

Lampante Olive Oil

Lampante olive oil has a sensory defect intensity higher than 3.5 and an acidity higher than 3.3%. These virgin olive oils cannot be consumed in this state and must be refined in order to be marketed.

The commercial category "olive oil" (not to be confused with the name of the family) is actually a lampante olive oil that has been refined and later mixed with a certain amount of extra-virgin olive oil to give the desired color, flavor, and smell.

Olive Pomace Oil

Olive pomace oil is a by-product or residue of olive oil. During the first pressing or first extraction, the centrifuge separates solids from liquids, thus obtaining oil and pomace separately. Pomace will be pressed again, and an oil of lower quality will be extracted and sent to the refinery. This oil is sold under the commercial category of olive pomace oil. Olive growers use pomace as fertilizers.

POLYPHENOLS

Polyphenols refer to the range of phytochemicals in olive oil, natural products which help with oxidation. Research shows they have a multitude of positive health properties. They also contribute to the stability of the oil as well as bitterness and pungency. (See "Antioxidants")

PUNGENCY

Also known as pepperiness, pungency is a tactile sensation that is felt in the throat or at the back of the palate; it's a sort of intense tingling, depending on the oil. Pungency is a sign of quality and freshness; it is one of the three positive attributes which oil tasters measure at the tasting session. Generally, olives picked green produce more pungent oil, but some varieties have a higher polyphenol content, which gives more pungency.

Oleocanthal, a phenolic compound with antioxidant and anti-inflammatory properties present in olive oil, is largely responsible for the pungency of extra-virgin olive oil.

PREDIMED

PREDIMED is an acronym that stands for PREvention con DIeta MEDiterránea (Prevention by Mediterranean Diet), a group of Spanish researchers who carry out studies based on the Mediterranean diet.

REFINING

Refining refers to the chemical and physical processes which remove all the unpleasant characteristics of oil; these include colors, tastes, and odors. No refined oil can legally carry the "extra virgin" label.

Lampante virgin olive oil is not suitable for consumption, and it requires a refining process to remove any chemical or sensory flaws such as free fatty acids, odors, and other impurities. Unfortunately, this chemical process also destroys all the high nutritional value items, such as pigments that give color, volatile compounds, and polyphenols. Once refined, olive oil has no more color, smell, or taste.

Olive oils without the words "virgin" or "pressed" on the label are obtained with chemical processes.

Retro-olfaction or Retronasal Sensation

Retro-olfaction allows us to perceive the aromas of food once in the mouth. It is also referred to as retronasal or indirect olfaction. Retro means "backward" or "behind," and nasal refers to the nose. To understand retronasal sensations, you have to remember that the back of the mouth and nose are all connected via the retronasal passage; in other words, we carry the aroma into the nasal cavity from the mouth.

We can retronasally identify the volatile compounds in extra-virgin olive oil more easily from 28° C (82° F) onward. It's the increase in temperature of the oil in the mouth, together with the addition of saliva and air, that lets you better appreciate the aromas. When tasting olive oil, retro-olfaction allows the appreciation of new flavors and complements the sensory profile of olive oil.

Sensory Analysis (Sensory Evaluation)

Sensory analysis is an assessment of the organoleptic attributes of a product by human senses. The evaluation of olive oil involves taste, smell, and touch, but not sight. The color of olive oil does not tell you about the quality. That is why olive oil tasting glasses are blue. By doing this, the taster cannot see the contents and cannot be influenced by its color.

For virgin olive oil, tasting is done in parallel with the chemical analysis; both are necessary requirements before bottling can take place. Tasting evaluates the presence or absence of fruitiness, pungency, and bitterness. It allows the oil to be classified into three categories: extra virgin, virgin, and lampante. The analysis is performed by an olive oil tasting panel, a group of eight to twelve experts who follow the IOC protocol.

Currently, the human nose is the most efficient way to detect the palatability of a product or to check for sensory defects. Today, a more hedonistic approach to olive oil tasting is becoming more and more popular among consumers. They look more for pleasure, harmony, food and olive oil pairings, production know-how, and varieties of olives. And just as it is with wine, olive oil characteristics are very much appreciated in this new tasting style.

SHELF LIFE

Extra-virgin olive oil is a fresh product, and, consequently, it deteriorates with time. It loses its nutritional and aromatic qualities and oxidizes. Olive oil shelf life depends on how it is stored and the variety of olives used to make the oil. Shelf life can range from six to twenty-four months for varieties rich in polyphenols if they are stored under proper conditions.

It is important to protect extra-virgin olive oil from light, air, and wide temperature fluctuations, especially heat. It is best to consume a bottle within three to six months after opening.

TASTE

(See "Basic Tastes")

VARIETY

There are more than 1,740 varieties of olives in the world and lots more to be discovered. Just as different grapes create different flavors of wine, olive varieties give typical organoleptic, chemical, and agronomic character to the olive tree and its oil. Here are some of the best-known olive varieties: Picual from southern Spain, Picholine from France, Koroneiki from Greece, Coratina from Italy, and Chemlali from Tunisia.

REFERENCES

We have read and studied thousands of published scientific studies for this book and for our own interest. We cannot list them all here, but here are the references that have directly supported this book. They include the most useful medical and scientific data supporting the benefits of incorporating extra-virgin olive oil into our daily routine.

Part I

OLIVE OIL, THE CORNERSTONE OF MEDITERRANEAN HISTORY

Cardenas, Raphael, and Juan Vilar. *The International Olive Oil Production Sector: A Descriptive Study of the Different Producing Countries.* GEA Westfalia Separator Ibérica Centre for Excellence in Olive Oil: 2012.

"Olive Oil." Wikipedia.com. https://en.wikipedia.org/wiki/Olive_oil.

"Know Everything: History." Huiles-et-Olives.fr. http://huiles-et-olives.fr/en/know-everything/history/.

"L'Huile d'Olive." Adelirose.free.fr. http://adelirose.free.fr/dossier/aliments/huil_oliv.htm.

Barjol, Jean Louis. "L'économie mondiale de l'huile d'olive." *EDP Sciences*, 2014. http://www.ocl-journal.org/articles/ocl/pdf/2014/05/ocl140010.pdf.

M. Abdellatif Ghedira (the new International Olive Oil Council Executive Director, who was nominated in January 2016) in discussion with the author, February 2016.

Understanding Fats

"Actualisation des Apports Nutritionnels Conseillés pour les Acides Gras." ANSES, May 2011. https://www.anses.fr/fr/system/files/NUT2006sa0359Ra. pdf.

Anne-Laure Meunier (dietician nutritionist) in discussion with the author, November 2015. Lectures on nutrition and diet to EDNH (School of Dietetics and Human Nutrition) and the Courts of Paris Diderot. Coauthor of the book *Power, Nutrition and Plans* to Studyrama editions. http://www. annelauremeunier.com.

From Olive to Oil

Uceda, Marino, Aguilera Mari Paz, and Mazzucchelli Isabel. *Manual de Cata y Maridaje del Aceite de Oliva—Proceso de Elaboración: Del Árbol a la Bodega.* Almuzara: 2010. Pp. 23–45.

Juan M. Olivares (producer of olive oil) in discussion with the author during the harvesting time in Hellín, Spain. November 2015. Further information can be found at http://www.pagodepenarrubia.com/.

"Valorisation des Sous-Produits de l'Olivier." Fellah-trade.com. http://www. fellahtrade.com/fr/produire/conseil-technique/sous-produits-olivier.

"Huesos de Aceituna para Producir Alimentos Funcionales contra la Hipertensión o el Colesterol." Mercacei.com. March 2016. http://www.mercacei.com/ noticia/45298/Actualidad/huesos-aceituna-produciralimentos-funcionales-contra-hipertensi%C3%B3n-o-colesterol.html.

Part II

Wonder 1: Olive Oil Contains Oleocanthal, a Natural Anti-Inflammatory

Gimeno, Iván L. "Researcher to Share Details of 'Thrilling Discovery.'" *Olive Oil Times*, November 2014. http://www.oliveoiltimes.com/olive-oil-health-news/ beauchamp-shares-details-oleocanthal-discoverycordoba/42667.

"Olive Oil Reduces Arthritis Inflammation." *Arthritis Today Magazine*, January 2015. http://blog.arthritis.org/living-with-arthritis/ olive-oil-anti-inflammatory-arthritis-diet/.

Dr. Roberta Holt (University of California) in communication with authors. For further information from Dr. Holt, see http://www.oleocanthal.es/un-oceano-de-salud/.

Jose Antonio Amerigo (retired Spanish physician) and Daniel Garcia Peinado (chef in a restaurant in Málaga, Spain) in e-mail messages to authors, November 2015.

The Oleocanthal International Society: http://www.oleocanthal.es/oleocanthal-international-society/.

WONDER 2: OLIVE OIL COMBATS AND PREVENTS CANCER

Branson, Ken. "Ingredient in Olive Oil Looks Promising in the Fight Against Cancer." *Rutgers Today*, February 2015. http://news.rutgers.edu/research-news/ingredient-olive-oil-looks-promising-fight-against-cancer/20150211#.V8fN-bPtbUL.

Paul Breslin (professor in the Department of Nutritional Sciences at Rutgers University, a member at the Monell Chemical Senses Center, and adjunct professor in the Department of Anatomy and Cell Biology of the School of Dental Medicine at the University of Pennsylvania) in an e-mail message to authors, July 2015.

Oreste Gualillo (PharmD, PhD, head researcher at the NeuroEndocrine Interactions in Rheumatology and Inflammatory Diseases laboratory, Santiago University Clinical Hospital) in discussion with the author, March 2016.

"The Endocannabinoid System." *Fundación Canna*. http://www.fundacion-canna.es/en/endocannabinoid-system.

Mauro Maccorrone (professor at the University Campus Bio-Medico of Rome, Italy) in discussion with the author, May 2015.

Lee, Martin A. "Olive Oil, Cancer and the CB-1 Receptor." Projectcbd.org. November 2014. https://www.projectcbd.org/article/olive-oil-cancer-and-cb-1-receptor.

Filik, L., and O. Ozyilkan. "Olive-Oil Consumption and Cancer Risk." *European Journal of Clinical Nutrition* 57 (2003): 191. http://www.nature.com/ejcn/journal/v57/n1/full/1601497a.html

Newmark, HL. "Squalene, Olive Oil, and Cancer Risk: Review and Hypothesis." *Annals of the New York Academy of Sciences* 889 (1999): 193–203. http://www.ncbi.nlm.nih.gov/pubmed/10668494.

Trichopoulou, Antonia, Christina Bamia, Lagiou Pagona, and Dimitrios Trichopoulo. "Conformity to Traditional Mediterranean Diet and Breast Cancer Risk in the Greek EPIC (European Prospective Investigation into Cancer and Nutrition) Cohort." *American Society for Nutrition*, 2010. http://ajcn.nutrition.org/content/92/3/620.full.

Tjan, Lukas T. S. "Squalene: The Miraculous Essential Omega 2 Oil." Scienceforlife.eu. http://www.scienceforlife.eu/tekst%20what%20is%20squalenel.htm.

Martínez-González, Miguel A. "Mediterranean Diet Plus Olive Oil Associated with Reduced Breast Cancer Risk." JAMA Internal Medicine, September 2015. http://media.jamanetwork.com/newsitem/mediterranean-diet-plus-olive-oil-associated-with-reduced-breast-cancer-risk/.

Cancer Research UK: http://www.cancerresearchuk.org/health-professional/breast-cancerstatistics#heading-Zero.

Michelle Harvie (UK dietician) in discussion with the author, January 2016. For further information, see https://preventbreastcancer.org.uk/about-us/the-nightingale-centre/.

José Gaforio (Immunology Division, Department of Health Sciences, University of Jaén, Spain) in an e-mail message to the authors, July 2015.

Sánchez-Quesada C., A. López-Biedma, and José J. Gaforio. "Oleanolic Acid, a Compound Present in Grapes and Olives, Protects against Genotoxicity in Human Mammary Epithelial Cells." *Molecules* 20, no. 8 (2015): 13670–13688. http://www.mdpi.com/1420-3049/20/8/13670.

Moral, R., R. Escrich, M. Solanas, et al. "Diets High in Corn Oil or Extra-Virgin Olive Oil Differentially Modify the Gene Expression Profile of the Mammary Gland and Influence Experimental Breast Cancer Susceptibility." *European Journal of Nutrition* 55 (2015): 1397. http://link.springer.com/article/10.1007%2Fs00394-015-0958-2.

"Les Huiles Végétales de A à Z." Leshuilesvegetales.fr. http://www.leshuilesvegetales.fr/category/huiles-vegetales-a-z/.

WONDER 3: OLIVE OIL BEAUTIFIES, PROTECTS, AND REJUVENATES BEAUTIFUL SKIN

Alech, Alice. *An Olive Oil Tour of France: Revival of Savon de Marseille.* CreateSpace Independent Publishing Platform, 2012. P. 33. https://www.amazon.com/Olive-Oil-Tour-France/dp/1480208442.

Passion Savon: http://www.passion-savon.fr/en/.

"Squalane." Wikipedia.org. https://en.wikipedia.org/wiki/Squalane.

"Independent Research." Bloom. http://www.bloomassociation.org/en/
our-actions/our-activities/independant-research/.

Najmi, M., Z. Vahdat Shariatpanahi, M. Tolouei, and Z. Amiri. "Effect of Oral
Olive Oil on Healing of 10–20% Total Body Surface Area Burn Wounds in
Hospitalized Patients." *Burns* 41, no. 3 (2015): 493–496. http://www.ncbi.nlm.
nih.gov/pubmed/25306088.

Nia Hafsia (olive oil soap maker) in discussion with the author, 2016.

WONDER 4: OLIVE OIL KEEPS BONES HEALTHY

"DEXA (DXA) scan." Nhs.uk. http://www.nhs.uk/conditions/DEXA-scan/Pages/
Introduction.aspx.

Benetou, V., P. Orfanos, U. Pettersson-Kymmer, et al. "Mediterranean Diet and
Incidence of Hip Fractures in a European Cohort." *Osteoporosis International*
24, no. 5 (2013): 1587–1598. http://link.springer.com/article/10.1007/
s00198-012-2187-3.

Saleh, Nermine K., and Hanan A. Saleh. "Olive Oil Effectively Mitigates
Ovariectomy-Induced Osteoporosis in Rats." *BMC Complement Alternative
Med*, 2011. http://www.ncbi.nlm.nih.gov/pmc/articles/PMC3045997/.

Filip R., S. Possemiers, A. Heyerick, I. Pinheiro, G. Raszewski, M. J. Davicco, and
V. Coxam. "Twelve-Month Consumption of a Polyphenol Extract from Olive
(*Olea europaea*) in a Double Blind, Randomized Trial Increases Serum Total
Osteocalcin Levels and Improves Serum Lipid Profiles in Postmenopausal
Women with Osteopenia." *The Journal of Nutrition, Health, and Aging* 19, no.
1 (2015): 77–86. http://www.ncbi.nlm.nih.gov/pubmed/25560820.

Fernández-Real, José Manuel, Mónica Bulló, José Maria Moreno-Navarrete,
Wifredo Ricart, Emilio Ros, Ramon Estruch, and Jordi Salas-Salvadó. "A
Mediterranean Diet Enriched with Olive Oil Is Associated with Higher Serum
Total Osteocalcin Levels in Elderly Men at High Cardiovascular Risk." *The
Journal of Clinical Endocrinology and Metabolism* 97, no. 10 (2012): 3792–
3798. http://www.ncbi.nlm.nih.gov/pmc/articles/PMC3462931/.

Wonder 5: Olive Oil Slows Alzheimer's Disease

Amal Kaddoumi (PhD, Associate Professor of Pharmaceutics, Department of Basic Pharmaceutical Sciences, School of Pharmacy, The University of Louisiana at Monroe) in discussion and e-mail messages with the author, December 2015.

Abuznait, Alaa H., Hisham Qosa, Belnaser A. Busnena, Khalid A. El Sayed, and Amal Kaddoumi. "Olive-Oil-Derived Oleocanthal Enhances β-Amyloid Clearance as a Potential Neuroprotective Mechanism against Alzheimer's Disease: In Vitro and in Vivo Studies." *ACS Chemical Neuroscience* 4, no. 6 (2013): 973–982. http://pubs.acs.org/doi/abs/10.1021/cn400024q.

"About Alzheimer's Disease: Alzheimer's Basics." National Institute on Aging. https://www.nia.nih.gov/alzheimers/topics/alzheimers-basics.

Netburn, Deborah. "A Mediterranean Diet Could Protect Your Brain from Shrinking in Old Age." *Los Angeles Times*, October 2015. http://www.latimes.com/science/sciencenow/la-sci-sn-mediterranean-diet-brain-shrinkage-20151020-story.html.

Valls-Pedret, Cinta, Aleix Sala-Vila, Mercè Serra-Mir, Dolores Corella, Rafael de la Torre, Miguel Ángel Martínez-González, Elena H. Martínez-Lapiscina, Montserrat Fitó, Ana Pérez-Heras, Jordi Salas-Salvadó, Ramon Estruch, and Emilio Ros. "Mediterranean Diet and Age-Related Cognitive Decline." *JAMA Intern Med* 175, no. 7 (2015): 1094–1103. http://archinte.jamanetwork.com/article.aspx?articleid=2293082.

Rapaport, Lisa. "Mediterranean Diet with Olive Oil, Nuts Linked to Healthier Brain." Reuters.com, May 2015. http://www.reuters.com/article/us-brain-health-diet-idUSKBN0NW1PN20150511.

"Mediterranean Diet." Patient.info. http://www.patient.co.uk/health/health-benefits-of-the-mediterranean-diet.

Alloush, Abed. "Greek Island Crete: Healthy Diet Key to Long Life." Eu.greekreporter.com, December 2013. http://eu.greekreporter.com/2013/12/18/greek-island-crete-healthy-diet-key-to-long-life/.

Fallon, Sally, and Mary G. Enig. *Nourishing Traditions: The Cookbook That Challenges Politically Correct Nutrition and the Diet Dictocrats*, 2nd Revised Edition. NewTrends Publishing Inc.: White Plains, MD, 2001.

WONDER 6: OLIVE OIL HELPS REDUCE THE RISK OF DIABETES

Sergio López and Francisco J. G. Muriana (scientists from the Institute of Fat in Seville, Spain) in an e-mail message to authors, April 2016.

"Diabetes." World Health Organization, June 2016. http://www.who.int/mediacentre/factsheets/fs312/en/.

Kenwright, Sarah. "Olive Oil May Offer Diabetes Protection." *Chemistry World*, April 2014. https://www.chemistryworld.com/research/olive-oil-may-offer-diabetes-protection/7252.article.

Guasch-Ferré, M., A. Hruby, J. Salas-Salvadó, M. A. Martínez-González, Q. Sun, W. C. Willett, F. B. Hu. "Olive Oil Consumption and Risk of Type 2 Diabetes in US Women." *The American Journal of Clinical Nutrition* 102, no. 2 (2015): 479–486. http://www.ncbi.nlm.nih.gov/pubmed/26156740.

Trichopoulou, Antonia, Tina Costacou, Christina Bamia, and Dimitrios Trichopoulos. "Adherence to a Mediterranean Diet and Survival in a Greek Population." *The New England Journal of Medicine* 348 (2003): 2599–2608. http://www.nejm.org/doi/full/10.1056/NEJMoa025039.

M. P. de Bock (author of "Olive (*Olea europaea* L.) Leaf Polyphenols Improve Insulin Sensitivity in Middle-Aged Overweight Men: A Randomized, Placebo-Controlled, Crossover Trial") in e-mail messages with the authors, April 2016. More information on his research can be found at http://journals.plos.org/plosone/article?id=10.1371/journal.pone.0057622.

"L'Industrie du Beurre Finance une Étude Scientifique pour en Redorer le Blason sur le Plan Sanitaire . . . C'est Raté." Nouvelobs.com, November 2015. http://tempsreel.nouvelobs.com/en-direct/a-chaud/6710-santeindustrie-beurre-finance-etude-scientifique-redorer.html.

Ferdman, Roberto A. "Study about Butter, Funded by Butter Industry, Finds That Butter Is Bad for You." *The Sydney Morning Herald*, August 2015. http://www.smh.com.au/national/health/study-about-butterfunded-by-butter-industry-finds-that-butter-is-bad-for-you-20150809-giuuia.html.

WONDER 7: OLIVE OIL HELPS REDUCE STROKES AND HEART ATTACKS

"Go Red for Women." American Heart Association. https://www.goredforwomen.org/.

Jordi Salas-Salvadó (author of "Olive Oil Intake and Risk of Cardiovascular Disease and Mortality in the PREDIMED Study," results published February 2014) in an e-mail message to the authors, 2015. More information on the research is at http://bmcmedicine.biomedcentral.com/ articles/10.1186/1741-7015-12-78.

Iannuzzi, Arcangelo, Egidio Celentano, Salvatore Panico, Rocco Galasso, Giuseppe Covetti, Lucia Sacchetti, Federica Zarrilli, Mario De Michele, and Paolo Rubba. "Dietary and Circulating Antioxidant Vitamins in Relation to Carotid Plaques in Middle-Aged Women." *The American Journal of Clinical Nutrition* 76 (2002): 582–587. http://ajcn.nutrition.org/content/76/3/582.full. pdf.

Dr. William Mullen (main researcher of the study) in an e-mail message to the authors, February 2016.

"Regular Consumption of Olive Oil Can Improve Heart Health." University of Glasgow, November 2014. http://www.gla.ac.uk/research/news/2014archive/ headline_376522_en.html.

"DMU Research on 'Healthiest' Cooking Oils Revealed on BBC's *Trust Me, I'm a Doctor.*" De Montfort University Leicester, July 2015. http://www.dmu. ac.uk/about-dmu/news/2015/july/dmu-research-on-healthiest-cooking-oils- revealed-on-bbcs-trust-me-im-a-doctor.aspx.

Hoffman, Richard, and Mariette Gerber. "Dietary Surveys and Nutritional Epidemiology: Can Rapeseed Oil Replace Olive Oil as Part of a Mediterranean- Style Diet?" *British Journal of Nutrition* 112, no. 11 (2014): 1882–1895. http:// www.ncbi.nlm.nih.gov/pubmed/25322908.

Pedersen, A., M. W. Baumstark, P. Marckmann, H. Gylling, and B. Sandström. "An Olive Oil–Rich Diet Results in Higher Concentrations of LDL Cholesterol and a Higher Number of LDL Subfraction Particles Than Rapeseed Oil and Sunflower Oil Diets." *Journal of Lipid Research* 41, no. 12 (2000): 1901–1911. http://www.ncbi.nlm.nih.gov/pubmed/11108723.

"Health and Olive Oil." The Olive Oil Source. http://www.oliveoilsource.com/ page/health-and-olive-oil.

Brackett, Robert E. "Letter Responding to Health Claim Petition Dated August 28, 2003: Monounsaturated Fatty Acids from Olive Oil and Coronary Heart Disease (Docket No 2003Q-0559)." US Food and Drug Administration,

November 2004. http://www.fda.gov/Food/IngredientsPackagingLabeling/
LabelingNutrition/ucmo72963.htm.

Gallego Edelfelt, Eric. "Stress oxydatif et antioxydants." *Olivae* 121 (2015): 31–34.
http://www.internationaloliveoil.org/store/view/101-olivae-121-english.

"Frying with Olive Oil." International Olive Oil Council. http://www.
internationaloliveoil.org/web/aa-ingles/oliveWorld/aceite3.html.

Part III

UNDERSTANDING THE LABEL AND BUYING EXTRA-VIRGIN

Granitto, Ylenia. "Police Uncover 7,000-Ton Olive Oil Fraud in Italy." *Olive Oil
Times*, December 2015. http://www.oliveoiltimes.com/olive-oil-business/
police-uncover-7000-ton-olive-oil-fraud-initaly/49929.

"Règlement d'Exécution (UE) No 1335/2013 de la Commission du 13 Décembre
2013 Modifiant le Règlement d'Exécution (UE) No 29/2012 Relatif aux
Normes de Commercialisation de l'Huile d'Olive." *Journal Officiel de l'Union
Européenne*, December 2013. http://eur-lex.europa.eu/LexUriServ/LexUriServ.
do?uri=OJ:L:2013:335:0014:0016:FR:PDF.

"Les Dénominations de Vente Autorisées pour l'Huile d'Olive au Stade
du Commerce de Détail." Afidol.org. http://afidol.org/commercant/
letiquette-et-les-mentions/.

"Huiles d'Olive: Des Améliorations sur l'Étiquetage." Economie.
gouv.fr, June 2014. http://www.economie.gouv.fr/dgccrf/
huiles-dolive-des-ameliorations-sur-letiquetage.

Pouyet, Brigitte, and Véronique Ollivier. "Réglementations sur l'Étiquetage et la
Présentation des Huiles d'Olive." *Oilseeds & Fats, Crops, and Lipids* 21, no. 5
(2014). http://www.ocl-journal.org/articles/ocl/pdf/2014/05/ocl140005.pdf.

"Olive Oil Cleared for Heart-Healthy Claim." WebMD Health
News, 2004. http://www.webmd.com/heart/news/20041101/
olive-oil-cleared-for-heart-healthy-claim.

"Olive Oil: Conditions of Competition between U.S. and Major Foreign
Supplier Industries." U.S. International Trade Commission. Investigation
No. 332-537, USITC Publication 4419, August 2013. https://www.usitc.gov/
publications/332/pub4419.pdf.

Mueller, Tom. "How to Buy Great Olive Oil." Truthinoliveoil.com. http://www. truthinoliveoil.com/great-oil/how-to-buy-great-olive-oil/.

"Recommendation Issued to Members by the IOC Council." International Olive Oil Council, 2014. http://www.internationaloliveoil.org/news/view/666-year-2014-news/516-recommendation-issued-to-members-by-the-ioc-council.

DIFFERENT CATEGORIES OF OLIVE OIL

"Designations and Definitions of Olive Oils." International Olive Oil Council. http://www.internationaloliveoil.org/estaticos/view/83-designations-and-definitions-of-olive-oils?lang=en_US.

"Olive Oil: Conditions of Competition between U.S. and Major Foreign Supplier Industries." U.S. International Trade Commission. Investigation No. 332-537, USITC Publication 4419, August 2013. https://www.usitc.gov/publications/332/pub4419.pdf.

Bushdid, C., L. Vosshall, et al. "Humans Can Discriminate More Than 1 Trillion Olfactory Stimuli." *Science* 343 (2014): 1370–1372. http://vosshall.rockefeller.edu/assets/file/BushdidScience2014.pdf.

"Testing methods." International Olive Oil Council, 2007–2015. http://www.internationaloliveoil.org/estaticos/view/224-testing-methods.

OLIVE OIL IN THE KITCHEN

Dra. Jessica del Pilar Ramírez Anaya and Dra. Cristina Samaniego (Pharmacy Department, University of Granada, Spain) in discussion with the author, February 2016.

Del Pilar Ramírez Anaya, Jessica. "Influencia de las Técnicas Culinarias sobre el Contenido de Polifenoles y Capacidad Antioxidante en Hortalizas de la Dieta Meiterránea (Phenols and the Antioxidant Capacity of Mediterranean Vegetables Prepared with Extra Virgin Olive Oil Using Different Domestic Cooking Techniques)." Doctoral thesis, Universidad de Granada, 2014. http://hera.ugr.es/tesisugr/22622457.pdf.

Uceda, Marino, Aguilera Mari Paz, and Mazzucchelli Isabel. *Manual de Cata y Maridaje del Aceite de Oliva—Proceso de Elaboración: Del Árbol a la Bodega.* Almuzara: 2010.

"Variedades de Olivo." Variedadesdeolivo.com. http://www.variedadesdeolivo. com/.

"Stratégie Mondiale pour l'Alimentation, l'Exercice Physique et la Santé." Organisation Mondiale de la Santé. http://www.who.int/dietphysicalactivity/ diet/fr/.

"Fritures, Huiles et Santé." Cerin.org, 2015. http://www.cerin.org/actualite-scientifique/fritures-huiles-et-sante.html.

CHARTS AND ILLUSTRATIONS

Barjol, Jean Louis. "L'économie mondiale de l'huile d'olive." EDP Sciences. 2014. http://www.ocl-journal.org/articles/ocl/pdf/2014/05/ocl140010.pdf

J.-L. Barjol : OCL 2014, 21(5) D502 Tableau 2. *Classement prévu en 2013/2014 des 10 premiers pays consommateurs d'huile d'olive et volumes consommés* (en milliers

Illustration "Consommation par personne/an" by Théo Gorjean. AFIDOL. http:// wesavoirfaire.com

WeSavoirFaire : Visites d'entreprises et Tourisme industriel. wesavoirfaire.com

WesavoirFaire vous souhaite la bienvenue en entreprise : Visites d'entreprises et Tourisme industriel en France. Faites du tourisme de savoir-faire.

Sundeep, Mishra. "Cooking Oils for Heart Health." Department of Cardiology, Sir Ganga Ram Hospital, New Delhi, India. February 2012. http://www. journalofpreventivecardiology.com/pdf/Issue3/Cooking%20oils%20for%20 heart%20health.pdf

"Mediterranean Diet." *Dietary Guidelines for Adults in Greece.* Ministry of Health and Welfare Supreme Scientific Health Council. 1999. http://www.nut.uoa.gr/ dietaryENG.html

Acknowledgments

Almost all of the data in this book comes from talking with the experts—researchers, growers, producers, nutritionists, and decision makers, all experts in their field. We are grateful for all the time they spent with us, for sharing knowledge and valuable insight. We could not rely only on publicized material for *7 Wonders*.

At the end of this book, we included a few simple, healthy recipes. We wanted to keep them short and invited only a few people to contribute. We thank all those who shared these gems.

We are grateful to Brooke Jorden for all her encouragement and support right from the beginning of our decision to write this book. Our editor, Lindsay Sandberg, guided us patiently and generously with her time; we thank her for her sharp editing of *The 7 Wonders of Olive Oil*. Special thanks also to our publishers and to all the team at Familius for their advice, help, and support. Without them, this book would not have been possible.

From Alice:

I am grateful to those who explained their medical conditions to me. They are all real people, though we've changed their names—from Joanna, who suffered from breast cancer and whom I met as a patient, to Susan, who spent time explaining her fears of the disease and what it is like to be an osteoporosis victim. We did not disclose their real names, for obvious reasons, but through them, we better understood the different diseases.

Thank you to the National Osteoporosis Society based in Manchester in the United Kingdom and to Genesis Breast Cancer Prevention, also in Manchester, for useful information, facts, and figures.

The researchers I contacted came from the United States, Italy, New Zealand, the UK, and Spain. Dr. Amal Kaddoumi from the United States and Dr. Mauro Maccorrone from Italy were particularly patient every time I bombarded them with more questions. I thank them for describing their studies in a way I could follow.

I am grateful to Janet Amos, the specialist nurse practitioner who filled me in on the seriousness of diabetes, explaining the challenges she faces working in a busy practice where almost all of her patients suffer from the disease.

Thank you to Nia Hafsia, a gifted and talented soap maker, for spending precious time explaining her work and the intricacies of healthy soap making.

I would like to thank all my friends and work colleagues for their inspiration and support during the writing of 7 Wonders.

From Cécile:

Thank you to the International Olive Council for allowing me to follow the training course in virgin olive oils tasting in 2014, and especially to Juliette Cayol, press officer, who was always available and responsive to our various queries and research information.

I am grateful to Mr. Abdellatif Ghedira, the new Executive Director of the International Olive Council, for taking time from his busy schedule to answer my questions.

Thank you to Sylvie Borrat Coirault, a pharmacy technician and herbalist, who very patiently helped me to understand the collective expert report "Updating the recommended dietary allowances for fatty acids" published in 2011 by ANSES, the French national agency for food safety and environment.

I am grateful to Anne-Laure Meunier, dietitian nutritionist, who works in Paris, for all her good advice on the Mediterranean diet and fatty acids.

Thank you to Juan Olivares, his family, and the Dominguez family for hosting me in October 2015 during the olive harvest in the olive grove of Pago de Peñarrubia in Hellín, Spain. I was able to follow for a week the harvesting time and observe the preparation of the mill before the reception of the olives for pressing. I recently had the chance to taste the first production of olive oil under the brand Pago de Peñarrubia. This was a very successful first production and excellent extra-virgin olive oil!

My special thanks also to Dr. Jessica del Pilar Ramírez Anaya for her thesis, "Phenols and the Antioxidant Capacity of Mediterranean Vegetables Prepared with Extra-Virgin Olive Oil Using Different Domestic Cooking Techniques," and to her thesis supervisor at the University of Granada in Spain, Dr. Cristina Sánchez Samaniego. This fascinating study gives us a new approach to the advantages of using extra-virgin olive oil in cooking, especially for frying.

ABOUT THE AUTHORS

ALICE ALECH is a writer and a qualified X-ray technologist (radiographer), specializing in mammography. She has worked and lived in France, the UK, Australia, and the West Indies. She discovered the wonderful world of olive oil when she moved to the South of France, to Provence—olive oil country—where the taste, flavor, and quality of olive oil are crucial. Drawn into olive oil culture, she has been covering olive oil news in France for many years, meeting olive growers, olive oil producers, and chefs—men and women who work hard and believe in what they are doing. It started a real thirst for more knowledge. With her health background, Alice was particularly interested to talk to the researchers studying the health benefits of extra-virgin olive oil. Alice feels strongly that a healthy, well-balanced diet can lower our risk of chronic disease.

Alice is the self-published author of *An Olive Oil Tour of France*, an appreciation of Provence's and Corsica's contributions to the world of olive oil.

CÉCILE LE GALLIARD comes from the north of France, where butter is traditionally used for cooking. After gaining a diploma in communication, she moved to Spain to continue her studies. This was where her olive oil education started, where she changed her cooking habits and became passionate about olive oil. Cécile Le Galliard is now a French expert in olive oil tasting. She is a recent graduate of the University of Jaén in Spain in virgin olive oil tasting. She was selected by The International Olive Council as the French candidate for the training and is now recognized as a skilled professional in her field. Cécile is a web journalist on www.jusdolive.fr and works as a consultant in olive oil, specializing in the creation of oil cellars, training, and olive oil tasting for professionals. Her olive oil blog, *Jus d'olive*, written in French, currently attracts 50,000 visitors per year. Today, Cécile is involved in olive oil training and promoting olive oil. She passed the Savantes Tasting Skills test in March 2016, an individual assessment, and is now a Savantes associate.

Cécile feels that the olive oil business is booming, and she is happy to continue learning more about the goodness and flavor of extra-virgin olive oil.

ABOUT FAMILIUS

VISIT OUR WEBSITE: www.familius.com

Join Our Family: There are lots of ways to connect with us! Subscribe to our newsletters at www.familius.com to receive uplifting daily inspiration, essays from our Pater Familius, a free ebook every month, and the first word on special discounts and Familius news.

Get Bulk Discounts: If you feel a few friends and family might benefit from what you've read, let us know and we'll be happy to provide you with quantity discounts. Simply email us at orders@familius.com.

Connect:
  www.facebook.com/paterfamilius
  @familiustalk, @paterfamilius1
  www.pinterest.com/familius

FAMILIUS

The most important work you ever do will be within the walls of your own home.

CPSIA information can be obtained
at www.ICGtesting.com
Printed in the USA
FSOW02n2211201016
26375FS